PREGNANCY
VIRGIN

PREGNANCY
VIRGIN

First time pregnant? Let's pop your cherry!

Mandy Mauloni

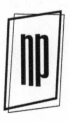

Published by Nightstand Press

PO Box 356
Katoomba, NSW, 2780

www.nightstandpress.com.au

First Edition © Mandy Mauloni, 2021

A catalogue record for this book is available from the National Library of Australia.

Title:	Pregnancy Virgin
Author:	Mauloni, Mandy
Subject:	Memoir, Pregnancy
ISBN:	978-0-6452762-0-6 (paperback)
	978-0-6452762-2-0 (epub)
	978-0-6452762-1-3 (mobi)
Cover Design:	Emma Bennetts
Cover Illustration:	Freepik

This book is for all the kids at school who asked about my inverted nipples ... may you spread the knowledge far and wide.

And this book is for my children, my greatest teachers even before you were born. Thank you for choosing me.

AUTHOR'S NOTE

This book is not a substitute for medical advice; it's a memoir based on my own personal research and opinions. It's been written primarily for entertainment purposes. You should always speak to a doctor if you have any concerns. Do not rely on the information in this book as medical guidance.

This book is not a doctor. This book will not shine a light into your ears, take your temperature, or touch your belly. Please consider your own unique set of circumstances and speak to your chosen care professional for medical queries.

Websites mentioned in this book may have updated their pages since the time of publication. I have no affiliations with the professionals and organisation quoted in this book. This is a true recollection, but some names have been changed to protect identities.

CONTENTS

FIRST TRIMESTER

SECOND TRIMESTER

THIRD TRIMESTER

AFTER THE BIRTH

PREFACE

This is a recount of all the highlights, lowlights and bits in between — from my orgasmic explosions to our baby's expulsion. There were so many times during my first pregnancy when I asked myself: *How did I not know this?* and *Is this really meant to be happening?* So, I decided to write down my responses to the tribulations I faced and the joys I experienced, in hope that one day, another first-timer might benefit from my confusion, my epiphanies, and my curiosity.

I'm not an obstetrician, nor a midwife, or even in the medical industry. But I am, and have always been, an organised person, a keen writer, and a person who likes details, particularly if those details are in relation to a quirky fact or an unexpected result — without a doubt, there's been no other time in my life I've felt so bombarded with quirky and unexpected happenings than during my pregnancy!

This is why I kept a journal throughout my first foray into the land of the breeders.

My first job after university was in journalism. I liked deadlines and I liked planning. My favourite reports were human-interest stories, especially those with happy connotations. So, in my mind, my pregnancy would be perfectly planned, and my baby would arrive right on time. I assumed that by being well-researched and organised, I could control how my pregnancy would play out. (In hindsight, this sounds rather insane ... but nonetheless, I was genuinely gobsmacked every time something unexpected happened!)

And I discovered that pregnancy doesn't roll the way you want it to, no matter how prepared you think you are.

Whether you're pregnant for the first time, trying to get pregnant, or have never been pregnant before and are simply curious about what pregnancy might entail, this book is for you. I hope you'll find it helpful to read about my experiences and those of my peers; I'll show you that none of your questions are silly, and I'll give you real-life examples from my own pregnancy, as well as share my research notes from the experts.

If you aren't an avid booklover, that's okay. If you don't know any pregnancy-related medical terminology, that's fine too. This book's written in simple language and won't take more than a few hours to read. (In fact, you can read it in less time than it takes some women to give birth!) There's even a handy Contents page so you can flip straight to the week or topic that interests you; there's no need to read my whole story from start to finish (although I hope some of you will). Each chapter is self-contained, but at the same time they each roll into one another to paint a picture of how my journey played out. There's also a 'Bump Box' at the end of each chapter designed to give you an extra boost of information or advice about a particular topic.

Make no mistake, this is not a comprehensive guide to 'all things pregnancy'. This book is an emotional journey that I wrote because I felt it would resonate with others.

While there's a chance that after reading this book you might walk away saying, 'I've got this pregnancy thing down like a pancake on Shrove Tuesday!' — more likely, given the varying nature of pregnancy, you'll be saying, 'Whoa! Who knew there were so many ingredients in a pancake!'

Within these pages, you'll find the answers to all the questions I didn't know I had, because I'd never been pregnant before. I researched, I asked the experts, and I spoke to my pregnant friends to gain a clearer perspective on everything from exercise to moving house while pregnant, from gender disappointment to feeling like you're losing your mind, from pregnancy massage to pregnancy yoga, from food cravings to labour, and all the other bits either side and in between.

In this modern age, I thought it would be simple to find the answers. But on the contrary, there was arguably too much information about pregnancy at my fingertips ... the internet had the information, social media told me how it was meant to look, and if I still didn't understand, there was 'an app for that'. It was confusing, and at times, overwhelming. I didn't want to be exposed to every possible pregnancy scenario; what I really wanted to hear about was authentic experiences.

This book helped me explore my feelings and my misconceptions about pregnancy, plus it filled a few gaps in my knowledge bucket about my anatomy — yes, even in my 30s, there was still plenty I didn't know about my body! Hopefully, this book will help you in similar ways.

People say, 'Oh, there's never a right time, darling!' and 'You'll never be prepared, my love!' but there was a little niggle inside telling me if I did my research and planned it properly, my pregnancy would be perfect. I would be prepared. It would roll smoothly. I would have the best pregnancy ever.

Here's how I thought the best pregnancy would look:

- I'd never know morning sickness.
- My skin would glow every day.
- My belly would be perfectly proportioned, and my

labour would be as strenuous as a heavy sigh.

- I'd diarise everything and research everything.
- I'd be careful about what I ate.
- I'd do the right sort, and amount, of exercise throughout the whole nine months.

I wanted to be the best possible mother, so that started with having the best pregnancy, right?

But the results were far from what I expected. In fact, if there was one takeaway I could give to all 'Pregnancy Virgins', it would be this: don't be upset if you can't cook the spaghetti; some days you're only meant to eat toast.

Or, in other words: throw the plan out the window.

FIRST TRIMESTER

WEEK 1
Befriending my vaginal mucus.

With the caution of a one-eyed surgeon, I stuck my fingers 'down there' and gently scraped around to find some discharge to study. I declared the day to be Clear, Watery Mucus Day. This was the kind of mucus that made a woman feel like she'd just wet her pants. You've never even thought about Clear, Watery Mucus Day before, have you? Because you secretly thought you'd just done a little wee in your undies, right?

I'd recently discovered that examining my discharge was a helpful way of ascertaining whether my body was fertile. Perhaps not the most *fun* way, but to someone as particular as myself, the process was very informative.

The vagina exploration was part of my 'warm-up period' for baby making. I was living on a diet primarily of fish and vegetables, and I had additional motivation to exercise. Vitamins were lined up along my kitchen bench like soldiers ready for battle. I'd been recording my visits from Aunty Flo for the past six months in a period-tracker app to establish my cycle pattern. I'd even asked my husband to give up beer for a month to optimise our chances of falling pregnant.

'My sperm needs beer to be in a good mood,' he replied. 'They won't swim if they're deprived of important nutrients.'

'Yeast, the main ingredient in beer, is not an important nutrient,' I replied.

'Your vagina contains yeast — case in point, that yeast infection you had last year.'

Damn.

Very shortly we were due to walk down the aisle, and immediately afterwards, we planned to try for a baby. As such, I'd decided to investigate methods of ascertaining my fertility.

What I discovered on pregnancy website www.babycenter. com.au (BabyCenter 1997–2021) blew. my. mind.

You know all that creamy, white discharge you find in your undies every now and then? Creamy White Discharge Day = glue for sperm. It's almost impossible for sperm to swim through this type of discharge and get to your ovaries.

I was 31 years old, and I had spent the best part of two decades trying to avoid being pregnant. How did I not know this about my body?!

If creamy white discharge is sperm glue, what does fertile mucus look like? I wondered. The helpful website article had photographs of real discharge smooshed onto real fingers. I initially found the images confronting, but then it hit me that re-enacting these photos would help me get a (somewhat greasy) grip on my own fertility.

Looking back down at my fingers and using my left hand to navigate the iPad, I learnt clear, watery mucus was the second-best type for conception, so not a bad day to get jiggy with it if I wanted to make a baby.

The Clear, Watery Mucus Day was supposed to be followed by Uncooked Egg White Day, around a day or two later. This was the clear, stretchy mucus that allowed the sperm to glide effortlessly through to my cervix around the time of ovulation, so this was the absolute best time to have sex in order to get pregnant.

Following ovulation, I'd be getting that thick, sticky white stuff, meaning it was probably too late to be trying to conceive (because: sperm glue.) One of the most important things I took away from the research was that not every woman goes through every mucus consistency every single cycle; some months I may not see some types of discharge. I just had to remember the most important one for getting pregnant was Uncooked Egg White Day. I can't say I'd ever been so interested in what was coming out of my vagina before; what was going in was usually much more exciting.

In hindsight, I suppose I *could* have bought one of those temperature-gauging ovulation kits, but I never thought of it at the time, and this whole discharge journey was pretty interesting.

And there was certainly no shortage of cervical mucus. During my very first gynaecologist visit, the doctor picked up the plastic speculum like a demon with a pitchfork, trawled around intensely, then pulled it out exclaiming, 'My, don't WE have a healthy amount of discharge!'

Ever since that doctor's visit, I've taken careful notice when thick, white mucus appeared on my undies, vaguely understanding that discharge had something to do with 'cleaning out' my body. But importantly, I now knew it was 'sperm glue' too.

I also knew my husband would be having Uncooked Egg White for breakfast on our honeymoon.

BUMP BOX:

Are you using a fertility app to plan your pregnancy?

I used a fertility app, among a variety of other tools in the lead-up to trying for a baby. But apps don't work for everyone — if you're planning for pregnancy and using a fertility app, it may be worth considering this:

In 2019, an Australian study (Costa 2019) short-listed 36 fertility apps that were marketed as being the most reliable in terms of efficacy and medical referencing. The research, by Eve Health Fertility in Brisbane in conjunction with Queensland Fertility Group, found a significant number of the short-listed apps made unrealistic and unsubstantiated claims. For example, some apps assumed all women had a 28-day cycle, and others didn't produce the correct ovulation date.

In fact, only 42 per cent of the short-listed apps accurately functioned the way they were supposed to.

With this information in mind, keeping track of your cycle is never a bad thing, but it's probably a good idea to exercise some caution (and additional methods) when using fertility apps to ascertain the best window for baby-making.

WEEK 2
What about morning sickness?

Trying for a baby was going to be totally fun, right? Sex on every surface, any time of the day or night. It would be like the Sex Olympics. I was going to shake off my inhibitions; there was never a better time to release my inner-Playboy Bunny!

On our honeymoon we spent most of our time in Cabo San Lucas, Mexico, a part of the world known for its distinctive rock formation called 'Lands End' and idyllic beaches. In Cabo, one of the primary sports (aside from sipping margaritas) is marlin fishing. With my husband being a keen fisherman, he made friends with other guests at our resort and was eager to hear their (most likely embellished) tales of catching mahi mahi, yellowtail ... and many-a-marlin. Then, before I could say 'Sex on the Beach', he'd talked me into a private charter boat — although I have zero interest in fishing, I have much interest in boat cruising.

We taxied down to the marina where we were greeted by our boat captain Ignatius and his skipper, Alex.

'Hola!' we both said (one more eagerly than the other).

'Hola!' Our Mexican captain held up an ancient brick of a mobile phone. 'I'm on da fon, see. Calling da feesh to find out where day be todeee.'

The captain and his skipper were pumped to the hilt and yelling out things to each other in Spanish; I couldn't understand a word of it. Husband was enthusiastically asking them lots of questions about fishing that I also didn't understand, so I tuned out as we set sail and watched the sun rising over the water.

HOLY SH*TBURGERS. My serene state was quickly obliterated. Why was the world suddenly out of focus? My husband was ex-navy, for goodness sake, with two experienced boat men ... couldn't they keep the damn boat upright?

'Geez, babe, are you okay?' Husband asked with a grimace.

Oh ... the boat was upright. I'd fallen off my sunbed, scrambled onto my knees, and was violently vomiting into the sea with rocket-fuelled propulsion. Long drips of saliva were hanging from my mouth; my breath was torturing my nose at every exhalation. 'Oh, just feeling a little off, honey.' I played it down. 'But don't worry — I'm sure as soon as the boat stops, I'll be fine. It happened so fast I didn't even know I was being sick.'

Despite their broken English, Ignatius and Alex must have understood the language very well indeed, because they proceeded to exchange amused looks with my husband.

'What is it?' I asked.

'This is *game fishing*, babe; the boat *doesn't* stop. It keeps moving ... the whole time.'

&^%! Followed by another extremely disgusting expletive ... I was glad we hadn't brought our swearing jar on holidays, lest it might have cracked under pressure. 'Seriously?'

'Stop looking around; focus on the floor of the boat,' Husband said. 'Otherwise find a fixed point on the shoreline and keep looking at it, and I promise you'll feel better.'

I tried, but I couldn't. I just couldn't. My stomach was

housing a small circus of acrobats. 'Need to lie down,' I mumbled.

'That's the worst thing you can do,' Husband warned. 'I've lived on boats before, trust me.'

But lying flat on my heaving stomach felt so much better, and it wasn't long before I fell asleep.

My limited knowledge of fishing includes knowing you use a rod, a hook, a line and a sinker, and sometimes you can use fish to catch other fish.

I woke from my slumber and started contributing to the fish hunt by hurling last night's seafood banquet into the ocean.

'We should turn back,' Husband said to Ignatius.

'No!' I yelled (well ... more like stammered in between explosions of food). 'When will you next get a chance to go marlin fishing?' I tried to swallow, but ... 'We're staying until you catch one.' I puked again as I said it, but I knew this was important to him. And it was our honeymoon, the perfect time to demonstrate how much I loved him, right? I clung to a nearby rope for dear life while Husband offered me water then grabbed my camera and took a few photos of me puking. I straightened my back and tied my hair up to at least try and look a bit elegant. *Side note: it's impossible to look good vomiting, even if you're posing on a private boat.*

Twenty seemingly-long (but in the scheme of things, mercifully-short) minutes later, Alex yelled to Husband to take a seat and grab one of the rods — we had a bite! I couldn't remember who the God of the Sea was (Titan or Neptune?), so I prayed to the Little Mermaid there was a marlin on the other end of that line, so we could get off this rocking Hell-on-a-Hull.

Ariel answered my prayers.

'You want to teek it to mount eet?' asked Ignatius. 'Or you can leeve eet wit us and we weel donate eet to zee cheeldren's hosepital.'

It turned out mounting a marlin and shipping it home to Australia would cost more than my university debt, so we agreed to donate it. (We had strong suspicions the donation would, in fact, be going to the Ignatius and Alex Tequila Fund, but hey, they had been good hosts.)

'Hola Meester and Meeses, ów was your feeshing trip?' asked the resort bellboy who had waved us off that morning.

'I was seasick the whole time, but at least he caught a marlin.'

'Oh seniorita, you must know zee treeeck. Beeg bar of chocolate on an empty stomeech, stop you from being seeeck on boat.'

Now he tells me. Goodness knows the number of times I'd eaten an entire block of chocolate on an empty stomach, but the one time I needed to, I didn't know I needed to. As I reflected on my bout of seasickness, I realised it must be what morning sickness felt like. *Wow.*

I thought about some of my girlfriends who'd had morning sickness every single day during their pregnancies. Sometimes *all day* ... for a whole nine months! *Nine days* of today would have been awful enough. So, the Sex Olympics wouldn't be held again any time soon if that was what being pregnant felt like.

But ... had we already taken out the gold?

BUMP BOX:
Strategies to combat morning sickness.

While I never physically vomited during my pregnancy, the thick nausea in my stomach often made me feel as though I was about to at any given moment.

The Healthy WA website (Healthy WA 2021) has an extensive and helpful list of tips for managing morning sickness, including:

- Stay hydrated
- Take ginger
- Eat small amounts of food often (aim for five to six Small meals a day)
- Chew your food well
- Get fresh air, sit outside in the garden and eat
- Practise relaxation techniques
- Wear loose clothing
- Rest after meals but avoid lying flat, and use pillows to raise your head and shoulders
- If you feel sick before getting up, snack on something like dry toast or salty crackers before you rise
- Take vitamin B6 supplements (10 to 25 mg three times a day), as this can reduce symptoms of mild to moderate nausea, and ask your doctor or midwife for

---

more information

- Do not skip meals. An empty stomach can make you nauseous
- Acupuncture, acupressure, and hypnosis are useful for some women
- Give up cigarettes and avoid cigarette smoke
- Do not take iron tablets unless prescribed by your doctor

There's an abundance of strategies online, far more than I can list in this book.

Please remember, if you're suffering, you aren't alone. Be kind to yourself and be sure to ask for help if you don't feel well.

WEEK 3
Will my pregnancy be like Mum's and Nan's?

I grew up in a small city on the coast of Central Queensland called Bundaberg. My family and I lived on a hobby farm with a cow, some chickens, a paddock full of chillies, and a ferocious German shepherd named Rex. My brother, sister and I had cow-dung fights, rode motorbikes, and learnt to drive an old Datsun 300 before we finished primary school. I didn't miss upmarket department stores like Myer or David Jones because I didn't even know they existed.

It was a steep learning curve, moving to a big city for university. Not just finding my way around the shops either; I had to learn how to drive on the M1 highway — and who'd have thunk it, there are lanes meant for fast cars and also lanes meant for slow cars! (I think I drove 60 kilometres per hour in the fast lane for about six months before I realised it was ME people were beeping their horns at.) But I fell in love with the Gold Coast. I discovered the beaches, rainforests, and fabulous nightlife, and from the get-go, I imagined myself raising children in this thriving city. (For the record, when I became pregnant, I was living one hour north of the 'GC' in Brisbane, but we had plans to move to the Gold Coast in the near future.)

Bundaberg was still an important part of my life, and I

needed to go back to have an important chat with my mother and grandmother. If I was going to become pregnant, I wanted to be better prepared than a Sushieze in a rice field. I'd heard (and my doctor subsequently confirmed) some conditions associated with pregnancy were hereditary: for example, morning sickness, big babies, and gestational diabetes might well be passed on, though not guaranteed to be. As such, I wanted to find out: what were my mother's and grandmother's pregnancies like?

'No dear, no trouble getting pregnant at all. Me gran had thirteen children, and she had no trouble, plus me mum had nine kids no trouble. Morning sickness? No, not a bit. Cravings? No, no cravings. Well, I wasn't overweight, so I didn't have to lose weight afterwards or anything like that. I was in better health when I was pregnant than when I wasn't pregnant. I felt very good the whole time.'

My nan also used to walk to school in the snow with no shoes on and bravely watched Second World War bombs go off from her bedroom in the little English town where she grew up. I could only pray any child of mine would have half her mettle.

'Me first one, your Uncle Brian, I had him on me own. Your grandfather was away with the army at the time. I had no doctor there and no stitches. I got up at quarter past three to go to the toilet and my waters broke on the floor. I gave birth alone. No, it wasn't scary; like I said, it was good.'

RESPECT.

'He was ten pounds and a quarter. My waters broke just after 3am, and he was born at eight o'clock. I think myself it's better to have a big baby than a small baby because they've got the strength to help themselves through the passage.'

Glancing down at my own passage area, I wasn't convinced

I wanted a ten-pound baby helping itself out of there. Babies weren't exactly known for their spatial awareness.

'You be sure to have your teeth checked. I was all right for Brian, but for Colin I had gum disease, meaning every time I cleaned my teeth, they bled like buggery, so the dentist took every single one of the teeth out.'

I remembered when I was a little kid and Nan once removed her dentures and scared the bejesus out of me, by clapping her bare gums together with rolled-in lips ... I made a mental note to make a dentist appointment.

'The best exercise I used to do was scrub and polish the floors. Now that's the best thing you can do for having a baby, get down on your hands and knees and stretch out like you're washing the floor. It's no good saying "Oh, I'm pregnant, I mustn't do this, and I mustn't do that" ... I used to take a five-mile walk every day and think nothing of it.

'In the olden days, they used to sit you on the potty to catch the afterbirth. It's like a big lump of liver, the afterbirth. With Colin and Shirley, the nurses wrapped the afterbirth up in a bit of newspaper and burnt it. And they used to wrap a bolster around you — that's like a long pillow — straight after you had the baby, for seven to ten days. You've got to pull your stomach muscles in, or else that's it. Nowadays you can get tights to suck it in for you; otherwise, you'll end up with a flabby belly.'

Mental note to purchase maternity control pants.

However, my mother has probably never worn control undies in her life; she was blessed with a figure like Olivia Newton-John.

'I didn't seem to have any issues losing weight after my first pregnancy. When I left the hospital, I fitted into a skirt suit I wore before I was pregnant. With you and your sister, I was more out and pointy, but with your brother, my stomach was flatter and round. After the first one, you're busy and always on the go. Some pregnant women lay around all day, and I think it's the worst thing for you. You've got to keep moving. I also had a lot of milk — I could have fed twins! I had to express it. The breast pads didn't do a good enough job; if I slept too long, I would leak, so I had to use your dad's hankies.

'When you were babies, we used to put methylated spirits on the umbilical cord. We also used talcum powder on you, but they don't do that anymore — something to do with breathing it into the baby's lungs. We used to lie you on your tummy, so if you were sick you wouldn't choke on the vomit, but you don't do that anymore either; you're supposed to lie babies on their backs. There are lots of things you don't do anymore.'

Based on this historical 'evidence', it sounded like my pregnancy would be a breeze.

- I'd feel so great I'd hardly know I was pregnant.
- I'd barely put on any weight.
- I'd give birth to the Incredible Hulk without breaking a sweat, and he'd virtually climb out of my vagina by himself.
- Thankfully, I would have plenty of milk to feed him.

BUMP BOX:

Speak to your female family members.

If you have the opportunity, have a conversation with other women in your family about their pregnancies and births. Did they have any issues? How did they feel about the experience overall?

While you may not have the same experiences they did, it might help put your mind at ease or even raise a question for your doctor you hadn't thought to ask before.

WEEK 4
How NOT to take a pregnancy test.

When taking a pregnancy test, exactly how early would you classify 'the first urine of the morning'? I'd woken every hour, wondering if I could take it.

2.00am passed. 3.00am passed.

By 4.30am, my patience was up. I nabbed the box of pregnancy tests from my bedside drawer, snuck into the bathroom and whipped out the stick.

My poor aim meant I ended up with urine all over my fingers. *Idiot!* Why hadn't I thought to grab a cup to wee in? This pregnancy business was already harder than I'd anticipated! For goodness sake, I couldn't even give my own urine directions, so surely, I'd struggle with a small child? Was I even emotionally, financially or mentally ready to be responsible for another human being?

After my initial shock, I managed to get some wee onto the stick, then shook it like a polaroid picture to help calm my nerves while I waited. I wasn't sure whether five days before my period was due was too early to test, but I was keen to find out.

I pondered how I'd tell Husband — assuming the test came back positive.

Should I literally bake a bun in our oven?

Nah. My face is an easier read than a *Where's Spot?* book, and I can't keep a secret any better than I can keep a goldfish alive, so I figured I'd just tell him straight off the bat. *(Fingers crossed, kids are easier than goldfish, huh?)*

Holy cow! Was that a second pink line on the stick? Well, it was, but it also wasn't. It was so faint, and I was so tired, maybe I was imagining it? I opened the test instructions, looking for clues.

Two little pink lines would yield more power than Jacinda Ardern and Beyoncé combined. What was that saying? *With great power comes great gains.* This could be the greatest gain of all. *This could change our lives forever,* I thought.

Damn! The instructions said to lay the stick flat after you peed on it — shaking the stick was not mentioned in the booklet anywhere. But would that really make a difference?

I picked up a second test stick to get some sort of confirmation, but damn — I didn't have enough urine left to last the required five seconds! It lasted more like two and a half. I lay the stick flat anyway, then closed my eyes and strained my bladder in search of more urine ... with no luck. When I opened my eyes and looked down, I saw a second pink line on that test too ... but it was also so pale, it was barely even there.

I'd done the test incorrectly both times. They could be two false positives.

But what were the chances of two false positives? Now I wasn't just out of pee, I was also out of pregnancy tests.

Desperate for a second opinion, I took my first test back to the bedroom. But should I really show Husband, or try to keep it a secret until I knew for sure?

'Where have you been?' he murmured with his eyes still closed.

'I had to let Captain outside for a wee,' I lied. 'He was pawing at the door.' *Should I give away the secret?* I wondered. *Come on, you're not ASIO.* 'I also got a bit excited and did a pregnancy test.'

'At 4.30 in the morning? Babe. Geez. What did it say?'

'It's inconclusive. Can I turn on the lights and show you?'

'Now?'

Dead silence. I dead silenced him back.

'Okay then, let's take a look,' he conceded.

I turned on the light and stuck the stick in front of his face, holding my breath in anticipation. 'Can you see the second pink line?'

'Just.'

'I'm not even sure if I did the test right.'

'Oh.'

'Did you want to go back to sleep?'

'Yes.'

Really? You'd rather go back to sleep? You're not interested in talking about the possibility of being pregnant right now? I'm going to be thinking about it. In fact, I probably won't be able to think of anything else until I know either way. You're really going back to sleep?

But neither of us went back to sleep. Husband had to get up for work at 5.15am, and I spent the morning with my iPhone hidden under the sheets, looking at images for 'faint line pregnancy test' and reading forums about whether a faint line was a positive. (Apparently, it might be, or it might not be.)

I silently promised myself I wouldn't buy any more tests for at least two days. That should give the HCG hormone more time to build up. (According to the pamphlet inside the box, HCG, or human chorionic gonadotropin, was the hormone which, when raised to a certain level, indicated you were pregnant.) If I waited, perhaps the second line on the stick wouldn't be so faint — provided I was pregnant, of course. It would also negate the possibility of me waking up every hour on the hour again that night.

Of course, when I got off the bus to work, I virtually sprinted to the pharmacy and bought another three tests in case I messed it up again. I remembered being about ten years younger and sneaking around the pharmacy aisles ... thank goodness I wasn't pregnant back then; it would have made for a very different life indeed. None of that this time around, for I was as proud as a prostitute with a PhD when I handed the boxes over the counter and gave the girl a wide grin. 'Just back from my honeymoon,' I said, as though everyone wanted to know I'd been having rampant sex for the past three weeks.

'Congratulations,' said the sales assistant through thin lips.

'Thanks,' I said. *Yes, thank the nice lady for congratulating you on a honeymoon. Or was she congratulating you on potentially being pregnant? Or for having sex? Or getting married? Maybe her congratulations were actually sarcastic?* It was hard to tell, and I was so excited; my life could be about to change. I really wanted it to be tomorrow morning already, so I could try not to pee on my hand again.

'Have a nice day,' she replied, again in a deadpan manner, as she handed me a paper bag.

Yes, I sure will. I will have a nice day. It will be full of non-pregnant thoughts. I'm probably not even pregnant. What is the farthest thing from pregnancy I can possibly think about? Puppies ...? Nope. Umbrellas ...? Rain reminds me of sperm trying to push past an umbrella-like cervical cap. How about that bush? Which one? The one with branches the same length as your husband's ... forearm?

The next morning, I woke up at 5am.

'I better go check on the dog,' I whispered.

Leaving nothing to chance, I decided to pee in a cup this time — for accuracy — instead of over the bowl and remembered to lay the stick flat for three minutes. *Hum da dum. Just me here. Little old me taking a pregnancy test. No biggie.*

To be honest, we'd had so much sex on our honeymoon (and I knew from my discharge we were doing it at the right time) I'd be concerned if I wasn't pregnant. But it WAS still four days before my period was due, maybe it was too early ...

I checked the timer on my mobile phone, which seemed to be running slower than the postie at Christmas. *Why don't I use this time to choose some names? I like Cohen for a boy. Maybe Amelie for a girl. What about that Mexican mother who tried to name her baby Facebook? Is that masculine, feminine or gender-neutral? What about if we had twins ... there was the New Zealand couple who tried to name their babies Fish and Chips ... Wow. Two very clear pink lines.* I silently cheered. This was it. *Thank you!*

Then I snuck back into our room and ever-so-gently crawled into bed, hoping Husband had gone back to sleep, so I could surprise him when his alarm went off in three-and-a-half minutes.

'What did the pregnancy test say?'

'What are you talking about? I was just checking the dog.'

'What did it say?'

'That you're going to be a dad in June next year.'

'Really?'

'The second line was crystal clear this morning.'

'That's pretty exciting.'

We smiled at each other, and I tried to go back to sleep but with no success. I lay there and thought about just how lucky we were. It wasn't lost on me that there were so many couples out there who struggled to conceive. I was swimming in awe and gratitude to think we'd struck gold during Round One.

I then thought about all the foods I wasn't going to be able to eat for the next nine months. It would be a small price to pay, right?

All day I kept inspecting my body for changes. Weight = 56 kilograms, same as usual. Boobs = two tiny ones, same as usual. One day last week, I thought they felt a bit fuller, which could have been the case, given this recent turn of events. But my bra still fit me perfectly.

Stomach = bloated from last night's pasta, but I could still fit into my jeans, same as usual. Hair = unwashed and in a messy ponytail, no glossier than usual. Hips = ready for childbirth, same as usual.

It was surreal to think I was growing a human inside of me, yet I looked and felt no different.

So, yup. I was pregnant. And I had absolutely no idea what to do next.

'If you did three home pregnancy tests and they all came back positive, you're pregnant, honey.' The GP filling in for my regular doctor was a short woman who I guessed was in her early sixties, with short dark-brown hair streaked with grey.

'Does this mean I'm going to start throwing up soon?'

'Possibly at around six weeks. Tiredness is the big one, and often sore breasts, but everyone is different, of course. You'll need to consider whether you want to go public or private, which hospital you'd like the baby to be born in and which obstetrician you'll want to see.'

I'd had various friends who'd given birth at both public and private hospitals, and they had spoken highly of their experiences. But we had private health insurance, so we were going to use it. As far as obstetricians went, I had no idea who was supposed to be good — that was a question I'd simply never thought to ask anybody.

'You can have a look online at their profiles to help you decide,' the doctor suggested.

She took urine and blood samples to formally confirm I was pregnant, plus checked for any potential health issues that might affect my pregnancy. I was to pop back in two days time for the results and get a referral to my chosen obstetrician.

'Just be warned,' she said, 'if the obstetrician thinks they might be on holidays around your due date, they probably won't take you on. In addition, they only take on a certain number of new patients each month, and once they reach their quota … that's it. No more.'

I'd best get onto it then. Such a big decision. Who should I choose to deliver our most important package? Young or old? Male or female?

Husband pointed out that a female obstetrician would have probably been through childbirth, so they might have a more sensitive perspective — then conceded it was really that he couldn't handle the thought of a strange guy prodding around inside my vagina. He's old-fashioned like that. For his sake, I scrolled through some female obstetrician profiles, and one doctor stood out … for all the wrong reasons. Review after review were all about this obstetrician making mothers cry, forcing caesareans, speaking in a condescending tone. I wondered whether she'd ever looked herself up on the internet.

Yes, there were also some positive reviews, but the negative ones were enough to depress a Disneyland volunteer. I'd never have considered I'd need to research an obstetrician before choosing one, but now I certainly felt compelled to.

After a bit of searching, I found a doctor who looked friendly and, as far as I could tell, had terrific reviews, so I rang her office straight away and locked her in. Tick ☑

This was a secret we really didn't want to share with the world yet. It was a warm and fuzzy feeling having something between just Husband and me for the time being, plus given it was such an early stage, I was concerned I might miscarry.

Nonetheless, all day at work I daydreamed about baby names, and each time I thought of a good one, I'd be desperate to lean over to my work-wife Clara and ask, 'Isn't Camille a beautiful name for a girl?'

Two days later, I was back at the doctor for the results of my blood and urine tests. Up flashed 'Four weeks pregnant' in big red letters on her computer screen and I got a little flutter in my tummy. *Sh*t, it's officially real. We're making a human.*

The doctor recommended I make my first obstetrician appointment for when I was about eight weeks pregnant, and I felt very smug indeed at having already done so. Tick ☑ This pregnancy stuff was going to be easy-breezy! I was going to be amazing at this!

But just as I started dancing around the totem pole with glee, I found out the first of many things that confused me about being pregnant: when you are *eight weeks* pregnant, you are really *six weeks* pregnant. Yes — you read that correctly.

BUMP BOX:
How far along are you?

Now I shall try to explain one of the most baffling mathematical equations in the history of human existence (in my opinion).

Here's the deal:

Some very smart medical people calculate your baby's due date based on the first day of your last period. So, for example, the first day of my last period was 4th September. It was now 3rd October, so I was therefore classed as four weeks pregnant. However, I only ovulated two weeks ago and that's when the sperm and the egg met up for their sexy dance, so I could only be two weeks pregnant. In fact, I was two weeks pregnant. But doctors say I'm four weeks pregnant because ... because ...

So, I thought to myself, two more weeks until I'm 'six weeks pregnant'. That means in two weeks, I can expect the likely onset of nausea and vomiting. On the plus side, no more periods for a very long time (hurray!).

WEEK 5
Can I jump on a trampoline?

'Why aren't you drinking, Mands? Are you pregnant?'

When your friends know you so well that drinking ginger ale out of a wine glass isn't mildly convincing, you know you're in trouble.

'Maybe,' I replied, wondering whether there was any way I could hold off the news until I'd at least had my first scan and knew everything was okay. But I'm not a good liar. I was already worried about how I was going to keep up the illusion of the Tooth Fairy to my unborn child. 'It's a bit early to test yet,' I continued, not wanting to fib but also wanting to protect my secret for a bit longer. 'I'm not taking any chances, you know?'

'What do you mean, babe? When is it okay to test? How early can you test?' my friend Jaynie asked; she and her husband had been trying for a baby as well. (Another reason I didn't want to confirm or deny yet, as I was concerned news of our pregnancy may potentially upset her.)

'Um ... *not wanting to sound like I'd done hours of research on this exact issue * ... I think you can do it about two weeks after you ovulate.'

'You should test the day your period is due, if you don't get it,' another mamma-friend, Charlie, advised. 'Although I did, and it said I *wasn't* pregnant, so I went out drinking that night — and it turns out I was!'

Our conversation was interrupted by Charlie's four-year-old son, who wanted me to play on the trampoline with him.

'Mandy's got a sore knee, so she can't,' Charlie said over the top of me. She gave me a pointed look. 'Maybe you shouldn't be jumping on the trampoline if you're — you know,' she whispered, glancing at my stomach.

Phew, lucky she said something ... can a baby be born with a flat top after repeatedly smashing against the roof of a uterus?

'Jumping on a trampoline won't harm your baby ... well, unless you fall off said trampoline and land on your belly,' my midwife friend Samille assured me. 'Though as your baby grows, keep in mind that this extra weight will put pressure on your pelvic floor. You can keep exercising until you feel uncomfortable, or until your doctor or midwife says otherwise.'

'I got you a surprise today,' said Husband, grinning broadly.

'Oh, honey, that's so nice. I could use a little pick-me-up.'

'I bought you our very first pack of disposable nappies, and some baby wipes,' he said with a flourish and swung his arms out from behind his back with a big smile.

What a sweet thing to do. But where's the Ben and Jerry's?

'And we should also work out what kind of baby formula you might want to use, just in case, so I can buy it.'

No, No, No! This was a disaster. These baby preparations were making all the worst-case scenarios run through my head.

I was worried we were jinxing things by being too prepared. We hadn't even had the first scan yet. What if the baby was stillborn? I'd heard on the radio only that morning six stillborn babies were born in Australia each day. Six per day. How absolutely devastating. I couldn't even begin to fathom how people managed a travesty like that; in my eyes they were super-human. This huge responsibility floating around in my uterus was starting to freak me out.

As was the looming water-shortage crisis.

I'd heard somewhere that fresh water on Earth could start running out as early as 2030, and I was certain it had something to do with the pregnant women using it all up.

Obviously, I knew it would be thirsty work to make another human, but *geez*. Several times a night I would wake up with a dry mouth. I'd gulp a glass of water, then all the water obviously had to come out the other end too. Sleep, drink, pee. Sleep, drink, pee. And it usually took me ages to get back to sleep because I couldn't stop thinking about being pregnant. (Pregnancy insomnia — the struggle is real.)

Due to the lack of sleep, each morning I'd wake with about as much energy as a wet doona. All my motivation to exercise would go out the window. I was probably going to be one of those pregnant ladies whose additional bodily fluid content would be dispersed predominantly around my neck, knees and ankles, and my baby bump would join seamlessly with my bottom. *But that would be okay*, I told myself. *This may not be how you planned it, but don't stress. Even if you morph into Jabba the Hut, thus far you have a healthy baby.*

In all honestly though, I was a bit upset ... I was supposed to be doing regular exercise! I'd just have to make sure everything else relating to my pregnancy went perfectly.

BUMP BOX:
What exercise can I do during pregnancy?

The Royal Australian and New Zealand College of Obstetricians and Gynaecologists (RANZCOG) website is an absolute treasure-trove of information for pregnant women. Here's some helpful advice I found regarding exercise (RANZCOG 2016).

General Considerations for Exercise During Pregnancy:
- *Include a gradual warm-up and slow and sustained cool-down with each session.*
- *Avoid exercising in high temperatures and humidity, ensure adequate hydration and wear loose-fitting clothing.*
- *Avoid activities with the possibility of falling (i.e. horse riding, skiing) or impact trauma to the abdomen (i.e. certain team sports games).*
- *Take care with weight-bearing exercise and activities involving frequent changes in direction (i.e. court sports) due to increased risk of injury and changes in balance.*
- *Reduce inactive behaviour: minimise the amount of time spent in prolonged sitting, and break up long periods of sitting as often as possible.*
- *Perform regular exercises to strengthen the pelvic floor muscles. Avoid activities that add extra load to the pelvic floor (i.e. jumping or bouncing).*

In my opinion, pelvic floor exercises should be taught at high school. I'd barely even heard of 'Kegels' before I fell pregnant, and then suddenly when my pelvic floor was already under the pressure of a baby, I needed to make these muscles extra strong? Incontinence following childbirth is a real thing, so please don't underestimate the importance of pelvic floor exercises.

WEEK 6
How can I possibly be this tired?

Once I hit my sixth week of pregnancy, I realised any tiredness
I'd been feeling previously was, incredibly, almost unbelievably,
quite insignificant compared to what I was feeling now. I'd
wake throughout the night with either hot flushes or cold chills,
and the next morning it was like someone had picked up a
vacuum and stuck it down my throat, sucking the life and soul
out of me.

According to my doctor, this was morning sickness — just
not as I knew it. There was no vomiting for me. Just exhaustion
so powerful I no longer felt like myself. I'd expected to have a
quick morning spew and be off on my merry way, not
experience hot and cold flushes all night, and then wake up so
exhausted I was unable to carry out simple physical functions
like standing up for more than a minute at a time.

One day, I woke at 6am and couldn't get out of bed until
10am. By 10am I was feeling fine and guilty about not going to
work. I wasn't ready to divulge my pregnancy yet, so there was
no reasonable way to explain an absence to my bosses and
colleagues, especially given I'd seemed well the day before. The
fear of them thinking I was lying about being sick, made me
feel sick all over again. So, I went into work.

These flushes and chills repeated themselves, and every morning I felt so tired I broke down and bawled like a baby before dragging myself into the office.

Exhausted, anxious, insanely thirsty — I couldn't believe this was only my first six weeks of pregnancy. This was not how I imagined it. I was meant to be glowing from the inside, with people staring at me knowing something was different, but not being able to figure out exactly what. Instead, I was sure people were staring at me and wondering why I looked so awful.

BUMP BOX:
More than tired.

Pregnant me: *I'm so tired, and I haven't even done anything today except watch TV and go to the toilet. I'm going to bed.*
Partner: *It's only quarter past seven?*
Pregnant me: *I know.*
Partner: *... AM?*
Pregnant me: *What's your point?*

WEEK 7
When should I tell my boss I'm pregnant?

Suddenly, something crazy happened ...

I felt fine. Better than fine, even. I woke up feeling *awake*. In fact, I felt great. *IT'S SO WONDERFUL TO BE ALIVE!*

Naturally, the first thing I did was panic. Was I still even pregnant? My baby must have stopped growing, I was sure of it. I was scared that he/she may no longer have a heartbeat. I grabbed my boobs — not even remotely sore. *Faaark.*

With my first scan still another couple of weeks away, what was I to do? I desperately prayed to the Lord, the Pregnancy Gods, Ariel — any entity I could think of — to make me feel like crap again tomorrow. *Please, please don't let this be the beginning of the end ...*

After three days of no pregnancy symptoms whatsoever and panic enslaving my entire being, I discovered my worries were premature. Slithering out of bed to eat my Weet-Bix, I was then forced to lie back down from the sheer strain of lifting my spoon to my mouth.

My brain attempted to fire through the fatigue. Must. Go. To. Work ... Need. Job ... Must. Afford. Food. And. Cute. Rompers. I looked at my mobile phone, which was on the floor beside my bed. 7.20am. That meant I had forty minutes to shower, dress, drive to the office and slot myself into the 8am meeting. *Not impossible.* I just needed some stronger motivation. I opened my bedside drawer to grab the syringe of adrenalin, so I could stab myself in the chest like Uma Thurman in *Pulp Fiction.*

Hmm ... since I couldn't find it, I disappointingly conceded my current state of suffering was really happening. I was not a rich, sexy actress just pretending this was happening, so I needed to sort my sh*t out very quickly.

Sidenote: when you're seven weeks pregnant, some research on the internet may inform you your baby is about the size of a tadpole. And on this particular day, I decided I wanted to be reincarnated as a tadpole because I was already not dealing. While I was lucky enough to avoid vomiting throughout my pregnancy, waking up each morning feeling as though I'd just stumbled off a long-haul flight from Bucharest wasn't much fun either. In fact, 'waking up' is a glorified description; it was more like 'a small step up from being asleep'.

Tadpoles, on the other hand, function perfectly well with very little sleep. In fact, they only sleep when they feel safe, which I certainly did *not* feel, especially given I was now twenty minutes late to work.

Tadpoles aside, it was not a good day for me to arrive late. It was a frantic day of deadline after deadline, phone call after phone call, with no time to read the newspaper like every good media worker should, or even make a cup of tea. There were intervals throughout the day when I honestly thought I was going to faint because I needed to eat and there simply wasn't time. It was one of those Fridays when everyone wanted a piece of my boss, and we were fielding more enquiries than Taylor Swift at a Blue Light Disco.

I arrived home just after 7pm and my tank was sucked dry — physically, mentally and spiritually. Fast forward 48 hours to Sunday evening, and I was beside myself with angst. Despite doing nothing but read/watch television/nap for an entire two days, there still wasn't an ounce of energy available in my body. I physically couldn't go back to work. I would sooner die. Even going to the toilet drained me, and I don't mean in the literal sense.

Monday morning came and went. I knew I had to muster the strength to see my doctor again, stat.

'The worst of it will hopefully be over after the first 12 weeks,' said the doctor. 'There are no guarantees. Some women are sick throughout their pregnancy. It's up to you, Mandy, but if you're having trouble with the symptoms, I don't see any real need to keep your pregnancy a secret from your boss; you'll find most people are supportive. I'd like you to have a couple of weeks off — I can just say "medical condition" on the certificate, or I can say "pregnancy issues" — it's up to you.'

'Well, I'd feel a bit awkward being coy about why I was having two weeks off now, and then in another few weeks time saying, hey, by the way, I'm pregnant!' I replied. 'That seems dishonest.'

My doctor also suspected my exhaustion levels were at least partially due to chronic fatigue syndrome, which I'd been diagnosed with three years earlier. After suffering severe symptoms for the first twelve months, I'd believed I was CFS-free ... up until now.

To make matters worse, I'd been making a few not-so-little mistakes at work. I was honestly working so hard, I was trying my absolute best, but the tiredness seemed to be affecting me. It was confusing for me, and no doubt frustrating for my boss, because I thought I was doing everything right. Nothing made sense; the brain fog was acute. It was my professional reputation on the line, and I felt like there was no way out.

I wanted to quit work then and there, but I had to be realistic — my maternity leave benefits didn't kick in for another five months. And one of the perks of my job was the maternity leave entitlement, so there was no way I was going to give that up.

But, like many women who are in their earlier stages of pregnancy, I absolutely needed a break.

I felt guilty about taking two weeks off work, but it was 100 per cent the right call. I slept for twelve hours a night and napped one-to-two hours each day. Inside though, I was mildly devastated. This was not how I'd planned things. I was meant to be a strong and capable woman, who would smash all her career goals while growing a child. I didn't see anyone else needing two weeks off work, so why did I? I felt like a failure, and my mind was a mess.

To make matters worse, it wasn't just my mind that was a mess ... every day my undies were filling with enough mucus to drown a small rodent. It was like nothing I'd seen before.

According to the Pregnancy, Birth and Baby website (Pregnancy, Birth and Baby 2020):

Almost all women have more vaginal discharge in pregnancy. This is quite normal and happens for a few reasons. During pregnancy, the cervix (neck of the womb) and vaginal walls get softer, and discharge increases to help prevent any infections travelling up from the vagina to the womb. Increased levels of the hormone progesterone can also make you produce more fluid.

Increased discharge is a normal part of pregnancy, but it's important to keep an eye on it and tell your doctor or midwife if it changes in any way.

At least my discharge was working hard, even though the rest of me couldn't.

BUMP BOX:
Can I take time off work during my pregnancy?

Rules pertaining to this are governed under Australian Law, and the good news is, there's a range of entitlements available for pregnant women in the workforce.

The Fair Work Australia website (© Fair Work Ombudsman 2009) says: *'Pregnancy is not considered an illness or injury; however, if a woman experiences a pregnancy-related illness or injury, sick leave can be taken.'*

(This was the option I took — using my sick leave.)

The website also stipulates there's something called 'special maternity leave':

Special maternity leave:

A pregnant employee who is eligible for unpaid parental leave can take unpaid special maternity leave if:

- *she has a pregnancy-related illness, or*
- *if:*
  - *she has been pregnant;*
  - *her pregnancy ends after at least 12 weeks because of a miscarriage or termination;*

---

o *the infant isn't stillborn.* (See below stillborn
   information for explanation on this.)

If an employee takes special maternity leave because of a pregnancy-related illness, the leave will end when the pregnancy or illness ends, whichever is earlier. If she takes leave because of a miscarriage or termination, it can continue until she is fit for work.

While the employee won't be entitled to take special maternity leave if the infant is stillborn, she may still be entitled to take unpaid parental leave. Special maternity leave won't reduce the amount of unpaid parental leave that an employee can take.

While the 'special maternity leave' may not help pay your bills, it does give you the option to prioritise rest during what might be a difficult time health-wise, so it's worth considering.

WEEK 8
Why am I struggling to eat healthily?

At eight weeks along, I didn't look pregnant by any stretch of the imagination; however, when I tapped my lower belly, it felt firmer than usual. It was a very nice feeling; a confirmation of life. And while I hadn't yet put on a milligram of weight, I was consuming food at the rate of a sumo wrestler given an AAA pass to Sizzler.

Due to my pregnancy, I had a smaller range of 'safe food' options, and it rattled me. It felt like there were only about five foods I was allowed to eat — three of them made me nauseous, one I'd suddenly developed an aversion to because of the smell, and a salad (hold the soft cheese and cold meats) didn't come close to filling me up.

My eating habits had rapidly deescalated from Attempted Gwyneth Paltrow status to Depressed Bridget Jones. Due to the potential risk of listeria, I avoided eating many of the healthier foods I used to eat, like raw fish sushi or chicken salad (I liked the ones with soft cheeses — it just wasn't the same without the cheese!).

In my mind, this left me with ... junk food. I used to eat a sausage roll maybe once or twice a year, but at eight weeks pregnant, I craved them *once or twice a week*, along with other bakery favourites, such as mini pizzas and thick white bread with dollopings of butter.

Pastry, butter, ice-cream, bread and cheese — my new food groups. Obviously, not an ideal meal plan. I felt guilty, certain every other pregnant woman was eating as though they lived in a food pyramid's wet dream. Interestingly, Kentucky Fried Chicken had also recently released their first boneless chicken pieces in Australia. For the first time, my fantasies involved a man with a funny little white beard and glasses; just call me Mandy Sanders.

BUMP BOX:

Food preparation and foods to avoid.

According to the RANZCOG website (RANZCOG 2020), food precautions are important during pregnancy to avoid potentially harmful bacteria and prevent exposure to disease such as toxoplasmosis and listeria, which can cause birth defects, miscarriage and stillbirth.

While cooking and pasteurisation can kill bacteria, the organisation lists some important tips to follow:

- *Avoid eating raw and undercooked meat (including deli meats).*
- *Avoid unpasteurised dairy products.*
- *Don't eat soft cheeses.*
- *Wash all fruits and vegetables before eating them.*
- *Wash hands, knives and cutting boards after handling uncooked foods.*
- *Avoid foods recalled for contamination.*
- *Avoid eating undercooked fish or shellfish.*

WEEK 9
Seeing baby for the first time.

Husband and I twiddled our thumbs for forty minutes after our designated appointment time, which we originally thought was a long stint in the waiting room — but as it turns out from subsequent appointments, it wasn't. Our obstetrician rarely ran on time because she was often up all night delivering babies; I guessed that was a reason her patients couldn't argue with.

Dr McDelivery (obviously not her real name, but I thought it was a good self-explanatory fake name) was an attractive woman in her forties with short brown hair and a deep laugh. The laughing bit was important to me; given she poked her hands inside women's private parts all day, I figured a sense of humour was a good thing.

Husband and I were both looking forward to the first scan. But nothing prepared us for the enormous jolt that seemed to crack through our whole beings when the computer screen came to life with a moving foetus. We both froze and stared in amazement and disbelief.

'Is it moving?' I squealed.

'Yes, look — he's putting on a show for us all, right on cue. See, he's waving that hand there ... and look, he's kicking his feet,' said the doctor.

It was so surreal to see for the very first time this little moving person that we'd made, and even more surreal that he/she was going nuts inside my tummy, and I couldn't feel a thing.

'When can you tell if it's a boy or girl?' asked Husband.

'Looking at this specific type of image, not until about 18 weeks, though if you're lucky, they can sometimes tell earlier. Would you like to listen to the heartbeat?'

'Yes, please!' we replied in unison.

It was like hearing the roar of rolling thunder; it didn't sound at all like the *ba-bom, ba-bom* of a regular human heartbeat at all.

Suddenly, the responsibility we were taking on hit me like a cricket bat to the face and tears started rolling down my cheeks. This was real. Up until this point, I hadn't fully let myself believe what was happening because I was so scared something might go wrong. (Which it still could, of course.)

I was overwhelmed and relieved and in absolute awe. There was also wonder, surprise, joy, and a myriad of other emotions I knew weren't just a result of my raging hormones. Seeing our baby move for the first time was one of the most memorable moments of our lives.

'His' heart rate was 174bpm — apparently 'fast-ish'.

'They say faster heartbeats are usually boys, and slower ones are usually girls,' Dr McDelivery said.

Husband and I grinned stupidly at each other, just because any piece of information about babies at this stage appeared to make us convulse with excitement.

'Well, boys definitely run in our family,' said Husband. 'We hardly have any girls on my side of the family at all.'

'Weeeeell, I wouldn't be too confident just yet,' Dr

McDelivery replied. 'That's what they say in Australia. When I worked in London, they always said faster heartbeats were girls and slower heartbeats were boys.'

As we looked at our baby, I felt with overwhelming confidence that being an obstetrician must be the best job in the world.

'Do you ever get sick of this?'

'Never.' Dr McDelivery smiled at me.

Then I got weighed. No noticeable weight gain yet despite my thickening waistline. The doctor gave me a few different referrals, two for scans at the sonographer and one for more blood tests to rule out potential nasties like thyroid issues and hepatitis B.

Our baby was 34.4mm long, and I was nine weeks and six days pregnant.

BUMP BOX:
When can find out baby's gender?

Non-Invasive Prenatal Testing (NIPT) is an optional blood test for the mother, which can be done before she is ten weeks pregnant.

Dr Belinda Maier, Strategic Midwifery Policy and Research Officer at the Queensland Nurses and Midwives Union, said it was a relatively new test that didn't qualify for Medicare rebates.

'NIPT tests for genetic or chromosomal abnormalities, which is why it can also reveal the sex of the baby,' Dr Maier said. 'It's a different test to "carrier screening", which is usually only done if there is a known family history of recessive gene abnormalities — for example, Huntington's disease — and parents want to know their risk of passing it on.

She said many parents found out their baby's sex during a routine development scan at around 20 weeks.

My husband and I were both desperate to know what we were having, but NIPT hadn't yet been made available, so we had to be patient. No doubt, some of you will be vacillating over whether to find out or not, so here are a few pros and cons to consider.

Why you might want to find out in advance:
- It's still a surprise — you just get the surprise earlier.
- It may be easier for people to buy you gifts.
- You can decide with more confidence on a name and nursery decor.
- If you were hoping for / expecting a particular sex and it's 'the other one', you'll have time to adjust.
- People will stop pestering you and trying to guess.

Why you might prefer to wait:
- You might enjoy the surprise more — delayed gratification!
- Finding out the sex is not 100% accurate.
- Pink and blue might not be your thing; you may love buying and receiving gender-neutral clothes.
- Once you go into labour, being able to find out the sex might provide additional motivation to get through the potential pain.

WEEK 10
Why injuring myself became a lot easier.

With the upcoming expense of a baby, we decided we needed to rent a different house. One where the landlord wouldn't put up our rent by fifty dollars per week every six months, as had been our current situation for the past year and a half. We'd been packing boxes for a few days when I'd started to notice a niggling pain in the right side of my lower back.

Husband and I went shopping for a new couch that day, and the more I walked around, the more it started to hurt. Then suddenly, the pain grew ten-fold with every step and a sharp stabbing feeling seared down my right leg. I didn't understand; I hadn't had any recent injuries and no history of back problems. The only thing I could put it down to was putting a few household items into cardboard boxes ... but I was 31 years old, not 81!

Husband helped me hobble back to his ute, and I adjusted the passenger seat horizontally to get myself comfortable. I then pleaded, 'I need a physio. NOW.'

Unsurprisingly, there weren't any physiotherapists taking new patients at 3.30 on a Saturday afternoon. However, *I needed to talk to someone* about my issue PRONTO. I had to have a solid, drawn-out whinge about how much pain I was in. My

46

back really hurt (Husband certainly wasn't giving me any sympathetic responses). And I was genuinely worried. *What the heck is going on? Am I going to be okay?* I researched symptoms and they paralleled the early stages of *Parkinson's disease*, which I knew was highly unlikely but also not impossible.

What was I to do?

I called the government — they get paid to care, and the 13 HEALTH phoneline is an excellent resource for all Queenslanders.

A nurse gave me this advice: 'It's not uncommon for a pregnant woman to experience back pain, my dear. What you're experiencing could have several different causes, including sciatica. All those pesky hormones are loosening up your bits and pieces down south, getting them ready to try and fit a baby through, so injuring yourself becomes very easy. It's all part of the effects pregnancy hormones can have on your muscles and joints. Nothing to worry about at all, I'd just take a Panadol for the pain. If you're still having concerns in a couple of days, then you might like to book in with a doctor.'

So, even though I wasn't carrying any extra weight yet, pregnancy was already killing my back. I really needed to be able to walk again before we had to move house. *What if I'm in too much pain to do the bond clean?*

BUMP BOX:
What numbers do I need to know?

It may not always be possible to contact your own doctor or midwife whenever you need to discuss an issue regarding your pregnancy. That's when phone services can be extremely helpful, and we're lucky to have several in Australia that cater for parents and expectant parents, including:

Pregnancy Birth and Baby Helpline: 1800 882 436
Perinatal Anxiety and Depression Australia (PANDA): 1300 726 306
National Breastfeeding Helpline: 1800 686 268
Healthdirect: 1800 022 222
13HEALTH (Queensland only): 13 43 25 84

In my opinion it's better not to sit there wondering; call an expert and have a chat.

WEEK 11
Dental hygiene needs to take centre stage.

Brushing my teeth was now a visual that would put a horror movie to shame. Watery blood outlined each tooth like a red frame, then dribbled down my chin. I really needed a check-up; I thought back to Nan and her dentures.

When my dentist told me failing to floss had been linked to miscarriage (though this was extremely rare), you could have knocked me flat with a toothpick. I doubled my flossing routine to twice daily and stocked up on new toothbrush heads for my electric toothbrush so I could change it every month. Neither of these activities were recommended by the dentist, just to be clear — it was probably unnecessary, but I was desperate for everything to be perfect, including my gums, and I was rocked by the dentist's revelation.

Fortunately, the Australian Dental Association put things into perspective, explaining the evidence indicating a link was inconclusive and I needn't stress about missing a morning floss.

'There has been research on the topic of dental health and infertility/miscarriage; however, the evidence at this time is not consistent nor robust enough to definitely come to the conclusion that poor dental health/gum disease can cause infertility or miscarriage,' the ADA told me.

As my pregnancy developed, so did my 'Pregnancy Radar'. I would stare at strangers, give sideways glances to colleagues, speak to friends on the phone, and secretly suspect that because of something they had said/done/worn, it meant they were pregnant too. I felt like the Nancy Drew of the Newly Pregnant. For example, my friend Harriet rang to say they had bought a three-bedroom apartment because they 'wanted more space' than their one-bedroom apartment offered. Hmmm ... they needed more room? They MUST be pregnant! I kept picking up my phone to text her and ask, then putting it down again. I didn't want to be nosey. But I really wanted to know if my hunch was right, or if I was simply suffering from pregnancy paranoia.

Another girl at the office, Penny, was wearing a suspiciously flowing dress. I whispered to Clara, 'Look, don't say anything in case she's not — but my hot tip is that Penny is pregnant. Just by looking at what she's wearing.'

Next, I started thinking about all the things I had ever said to pregnant women, and I realised the things were all WRONG. One time I met a woman who was just entering her second trimester and said, 'Wow, you don't even *look* pregnant!' which, Pregnancy Virgin me thought was a massive compliment about how fit she looked. In retrospect, the poor woman probably stressed out and wondered if her baby had stopped growing, or if it was weird that she wasn't showing yet.

Another thing I'd said to a girl I knew was, 'You were so skinny before, your body will *totally* bounce right back.' Seriously, that had come out of my mouth.

Now the tables had turned.

As I neared the end of my first trimester, what really got on my pregnancy-goat was when people told me, 'you look so full of energy'. This wouldn't have been a problem if I *did* feel energised, but the fact was I had all the get-up-and-go of a one-flippered walrus. All I wanted was a trailer-load of sympathy, and I'd have much preferred to hear, 'allow me to piggy-back you up those stairs'.

I stared at my growing tummy and jumped on the scales, looking down in disbelief. This pregnancy was exhausting me to a state of paralysis, causing me to walk with the grace of a constipated ibis, giving me vampire teeth, and all I'd gained was one freaking kilogram?

By this stage, I was crawling into bed by 7.30 each evening, or earlier. I was comforting myself with the knowledge that by next week I would be in my second trimester — which meant, according to various pregnancy websites, there was a good chance I'd feel more energetic.

Due to my decrease in energy, I was shunning virtually all invitations that involved activity after 6pm, with one exception. Husband and I had been invited to a Christmas party that Friday night and I really wanted to go. It was the end of year 'MeatMeet' party, a steak appreciation society coordinated by my cousins. This group visited different steak restaurants throughout the year, and for each restaurant, there were score cards under the categories of Food, Atmosphere, Toilet Cleanliness and Service. At the Christmas party, all the points were added up and a virtual trophy was awarded to the best steak restaurant in Brisbane.

The Christmas dinner was always the most fun, not just because of the cajoling around whether that year's winner was truly deserving, but also the game that we played — everyone brought along a meat-themed gift and, if you opened your gift after someone else, you had the option of stealing their gift and swapping it for yours. (Some people call this game 'Kris Kringle'.) There were meat thermometers, Barbie Mates, and all sorts of carnivorous delights up for the taking, and I didn't want to miss out. As a kid, I'd never shoplifted so much as a stick of gum, so this was as close to stealing as I was ever likely to get.

We left the party at a respectable hour, walking through our front door just after 11pm, but I paid the price for my over-exertion, as I couldn't move off the couch for the rest of the weekend ... with the exception of sitting up to the dinner table to use my newly acquired steak knives. And after dinner, I brushed and flossed. (Twice ... couldn't help myself.)

BUMP BOX:
When should I see a dentist?

When I emailed The Australian Dental Association (ADA) seeking information about any potential link between flossing and miscarriage, I also asked for some advice around what pregnant women should be doing to best look after their teeth and gums. The ADA said dental checks were a good idea both before becoming pregnant and in the second trimester.

High levels of hormones can increase blood flow to the gums during pregnancy. Inflammation of the gums and bleeding from the gums with toothbrushing can increase and occur more easily. Smaller amounts of dental plaque on the teeth can cause the gums to become inflamed and bleed, compared to when not pregnant.

When preparing to become pregnant, as well as the necessary checks required with a general medical practitioner, women should also have a dental examination to ensure their oral health is in a good position before entering pregnancy. If already pregnant, receiving dental examinations and treatment during pregnancy is safe to do so, with trimester two being the preferred timing in terms of comfort and development.

Pregnant women should continue to keep good oral hygiene throughout the pregnancy by brushing the teeth twice per day with a fluoride toothpaste as well as clean between the teeth daily, using floss or an interdental brush, for example.

The ADA also said women experiencing vomiting or reflux should look to avoid brushing their teeth straight afterwards (it is best to wait at least one hour), and while waiting to brush, drink water, or rinse the mouth with water or fluoride mouthwash. This is because brushing straight away may cause increased tooth wear.

WEEK 12
Sweet dreams are made of HCG.

I was standing at the edge of my bed when a man I didn't know — although strangely, I felt like I'd seen him before — forced me to the ground and ripped open my shirt like it had a serrated edge. He gave me a sensual, knowing smile, revealing a set of straight, white teeth, shining like a diamond bracelet. Oh, of course! He was the guy off the Gillette adverts, all stubble and dark floppy hair, with a sixpack you could grate cheese on. We had hard, fast and sweaty sex where he said a lot of things I didn't really understand but nonetheless made me feel like a Goddess, then I rolled over and told him, 'We have to break up. After all, I'm married and expecting a child with my husband.'

I remembered this dream in vivid detail, which was unusual because most of the time I was flat out remembering whether I'd dreamt the night before at all, let alone recalling who was in the dream and what we did. But during pregnancy, these super-clear, crazy, sexy dreams were popping into my subconscious all the time. Maybe it was due to those extra litres of blood that were apparently rushing around my vagina like a crowd of Christmas Eve shoppers?

During those first nine weeks of pregnancy, I dreamt about having sex with someone — sometimes my husband, sometimes not — at least two or three times a week. Around the same time, I received the following text from a fellow pregnant friend, Kaitlyn:

Had a weird dream last night. Sex with a stranger. Hot sex. Really life-like. Are you having these at all?

To which I replied: *Nope. You're a slut-face. *Pause* Just kidding. I'm having them too, babe. They're crazy, hey?*

Do you think I should tell Bohdi?

Would you want to know about them if you were him?

Yep. I would.

Would it help if you told him I was a slut, too?

He might think I'm keen for a threesome.

Uh-huh.

Gross!

Why wouldn't you want a threesome with me?

Really?

Come on, you know you want it.

Urgh. I hope I don't dream about you tonight.

In real life, I'd never get a look-in with the Gillette guy, but I tried to make a bit of an effort with my appearance. With all the changes happening to my body, I decided a new hairdo might be just what was needed to jumpstart some feel-good juju. I was going short.

My ponytails generally consisted of bumpy bunches of hair that resembled the Leaning Tower of Pisa by the end of the day. But I persisted in trying to do them, because I was convinced having my hair up made my face look thinner, and the alternative — blow-drying it out — apparently made my head look like a mushroom (according to Husband). In an attempt to find another solution, I decided to get all my long, specifically-wedding-grown hair cut off into a short, sleek bob.

'I had a client in here last week,' said Jemima, my hairdresser. 'And I wanted to smack him in the face with my hot irons. He said to me, "Why do women all get married, have babies, and then chop their hair off in quick succession? When a chick looks like a man, it pretty much guarantees a divorce."'

As I listened to Jemima's story, I reassured myself that this loser she was referring to would surely not be speaking for all Mankind.

Looking like a man indeed ... I swaggered out of the salon with my stylish new bob, feeling sexy, head high, as if to scream out my femininity still existed, and I even gave my hips an extra little swish when I walked.

'Are you okay? Did you hurt your ankle?' the male receptionist asked.

One of the positive aspects of crashing out by 7.30pm every night was that I was excused from cleaning up after dinner. I was fortunate enough to have a husband who loved to cook and was very good at it, so out of fairness, my job was to stack the dishwasher and wash up. But now, I was overtaken with FUMIS — Fuck Me I'm Shattered — an acronym I created because neither 'very tired' nor 'exhausted' properly explained the full extent of what I was feeling. (It rhymes with pumice, as in 'I used a pumice stone on my feet following the marathon, and all that running made me completely FUMISED.)

My evening FUMIS would start right after dinner with my face getting very hot, like it does when I'm really embarrassed.

Once my whole head was on fire, I'd start to get dizzy as though I was about to hyperventilate, and then any remaining energy from the day would rapidly drain away from my body. This would be followed by my body weakly falling onto the couch and curling into the foetal position, with me frequently letting out long wails that translated to 'oh my goodness, I feel so incredibly crap right now I need to make noises like I might actually be dying'.

I performed this FUMIS ritual every night from weeks nine to 13 of my first trimester. I was counting down the days until my second trimester — when apparently most women started feeling better.

Maybe if I stopped having so much sex in my dreams, I'd be a bit less FUMISED when I woke up in the mornings ...

BUMP BOX:

Why am I having crazy dreams?

The Parents website (Parents.com 2015) had the answer I was looking for on their website.

Yes, many women report having much more vivid and colourful dreams during pregnancy than they ever did before. This may be due to those wild hormonal fluctuations you're experiencing, which can make your emotions (even when you're sleeping) and your dreams more intense now. But a more likely explanation has to do with how well or deeply you're sleeping these days. Since pregnant women tend to wake more often through the night (as a result of being physically uncomfortable, needing to pee, or because the baby is moving) they experience several interrupted phases of REM sleep, which is when dreams occur. If you're awakened during the REM stage of sleep or just afterward, you're a lot more likely to remember your dreams, making them seem more vivid, colourful and real.

The article went on to say:

Some women even dream about their partner having sex with someone else, which stems from a need to feel assured that you will receive support from him after you become a mum.

I'd also dreamt about Husband having sex with someone else. I think it's fair to say at this point, we were having more sex while we were asleep than when we were awake.

WEEK 13
That wasn't the sex I was expecting ...

What do you do when your baby's sex isn't what you expected?

Our 13-week scan with the sonographer was something we'd been looking forward to, not just because it meant we'd be comfortable telling others we were pregnant, but also because we'd see our baby in more detail for the first time. After this scan, everything would seem more real. We'd been anticipating this day like dogs at the cattery door.

'Honestly, you can see quite a lot more of the baby in week 13, compared with week 12,' the sonographer said, congratulating us on managing to wait an extra week to have the scan. In fact, the credit needed to go to all the things we had been busy doing to move house, as opposed to our incredible patience, but we smiled politely like the little calmness gurus she assumed we were.

She moved the probe around my gelled-up belly. 'Oh my GOSH!' she exclaimed, loud enough to wake any nearby babies, one in my belly included. 'This NEVER happens.'

Umm ... What never happens?

Then we saw the sonographer grinning as though she'd just seen our baby solve a quadratic equation in sign language.

'What?' we begged.

'Your baby is in the *perfect* position for this scan. Usually, I have to get ladies to run up and down the hallway or do star jumps to try and convince their baby to move into a position even close to this. Look at those fingers, I can't believe how clearly we can see each finger and toe. You've got ten of each there. And see this clear section behind the neck? That's fluid, and in your case there's not much there at all. That's one of the things we measure to find out whether the baby may have Down syndrome, but yours is looking fine. Aaaand ... do you want to know the sex? I wouldn't normally say as much at a 13-week scan, but I'm sure I can tell with 85 to 90 per cent accuracy what you're having, because your baby is lying exactly right.'

'Yes!' Husband and I said unanimously.

'I would say you're having a girl. Now — we always leave room for error, but I'd be very confident to say yours is a girl, based on what I'm seeing on the screen now. You can see this white line along here, that's the pelvis, and you can usually tell the sex quite accurately by whether the line lies flat or whether it's at an angle.'

Ours was definitely lying flat.

The sonographer said, 'Congratulations!' and smiled brightly at me.

However, my immediate reaction wasn't happiness at all ... but *guilt*.

Which in turn made me feel ashamed. Here I was, falling pregnant easily with what looked like a healthy baby girl. And instead of being excited, I was slightly shocked and rather numb.

I'd been sure I was carrying a boy. Everyone told me they thought it was going to be a boy.

Being a girl myself, I remembered what my teenage years had been like. I assumed raising a girl would be difficult. What if we clashed? My assumption (whether correct or not) was that boys would be simpler to figure out, so having a boy first would be easier. Plus, as crazy as it sounds, I wasn't sure whether I was ready to share Husband with another female. I fully realise how pathetic this is … but would I get jealous with all his attention on her? I really did want a girl — at some stage — but in all honesty, I just wasn't mentally prepared for it happening *now*.

In contrast, Husband had been really, really hoping for a girl, but never imagined he'd get one. In the previous four generations of his family, only two females had been born and more than twenty males. Given his family history, everyone was pretty much resigned to the fact we were going to have a boy. He had grown up with one brother, no sisters, and was very much a 'man's man'. Aside from his mother, he'd had very few female influences in his life growing up, so this news was his dream come true.

While I sat there in shock, Husband's eyes started to well up. He was completely overcome with emotion. 'That's awesome,' he whispered. He was going to get the little princess he'd wished for. Then he started shedding tears; I'd never seen anything like it. I didn't know whether to comfort him, to look away, or to cry as well.

Now, of course I was over the moon our baby was healthy, and seeing my husband so happy did make me melt a little inside. But I did wonder … so many people I knew waited the whole nine months to find out the sex. Imagine if I'd waited nine months, been on the hospital bed, full of hormones, physically, emotionally and mentally exhausted, thinking I was pushing out a boy and then … while beside myself with pain, I found out it was a girl? Would I feel as shocked and numb as I felt now? I called it 'gender shock' — similarly called 'gender disappointment', but I didn't particularly identify with that term. To me, my daughter wasn't a disappointment … just unexpected.

I was struggling to get my head around it.

I suppose if you didn't have any thoughts either way on the gender, then you wouldn't mind waiting the whole nine months, but I was one of those souls who had to plan. Waiting out the entire pregnancy to find out whether we were having a boy or a girl was never an option for me, and thankfully, Husband wanted to know as early as possible too.

After Husband regained his composure, we listened to the baby's heartbeat; it was 154bpm.

'But it was over 170 a few weeks ago?' I queried.

'Don't worry, that's normal. Around the 10-week mark is as fast as it will get, then it starts to slow down from there,' said the sonographer.

Husband could tell from my demeanour that something was up.

So, I blurted out, 'Didn't you want to have a boy first, so he could look after the girl?'

Now, before every feminist reading this book starts yelling at me, I'm fully aware I'd fallen into the trap of gender stereotyping in an age when we all know 'girls can do anything'. Why did I even think this question was okay to verbalise?

I don't know. Possibly because I grew up on a plentiful diet of Enid Blyton? But more than that — in retrospect, I believe this ignorant question was framed by my own personal strengths and weaknesses. I'm not confident using a hammer. I couldn't win a fight against a garden gnome. In the past, I've been guilty of flirting and/or playing dumb to get my own way. (Though perhaps the latter is a strength as opposed to a weakness; you've got to use what you've got.) I grew up with an older brother, and I have always believed males were the physically stronger sex.

It's not that I believe women can't be tough. And I as sure as eggs know they can be smarter. But in terms of the immense challenges facing children in the school environment — such as catching the bus, changing friendship groups, competitiveness in the playground, consent when they're older — I was worried about potentially having a daughter who struggled to defend herself.

In my mind, an older brother could help with some of those issues.

'Not at all,' Husband replied. 'Mandy, you know that when we have a little boy, I'd like him to have an older sister to help rub off some of my "blokey" influence on him and to give him a bit more of a female figure in his life. I didn't have that. I think having a girl first will be absolutely great.'

Oh. When you put it like that, it sounded ... well, I rather wanted to swoon over my husband talking about his feminine side. His point of view was the catalyst for me to stop worrying about whether I'd be able to manage raising a girl. For now, I decided to simply enjoy the fact we were having a beautiful little baby girl who, at least for the first 13 weeks of her life, was perfect. It wasn't lost on me that so many women had an incredibly difficult time conceiving, and here I was, pregnant first go and upset because the sex wasn't what I expected. I knew it was an ungrateful attitude, but I had no control over the thoughts entering my head.

We rang our family straight after the scan. Husband's parents were particularly overjoyed hearing it was going to be a girl, given their family history.

My nan was also excited. 'Oh, a girl!' she exclaimed. 'You know, when you're pregnant with a girl, you're big *all* the way around, not just your tummy like with a boy, but your bum and your hips as well. Congratulations, darling, that's wonderful news.'

BUMP BOX:
Gender disappointment.

Emma Black, a Queensland-based clinical psychologist, says gender disappointment isn't uncommon. Her website (Black 2020) advises three main strategies to cope with the related emotions:

1. Accept your feelings
Upon hearing the gender of your baby, you felt disappointed and sad, because the life you'd imagined is no longer a possibility. When there's a gap between what you want and what you have, this always causes some type of pain. Additionally, when you tell yourself you shouldn't feel the way you do, these feelings get bigger, hang around for longer than expected, or you need to escape or avoid them. Other negative feelings also emerge: you wind up feeling guilty and ashamed, because you should just be happy with what you've got. The negative feelings seem to grow, which doesn't help you process your disappointment.

One way to get out of this vicious cycle is to accept your feelings. Give yourself permission to feel sad or disappointed, even if you don't like feeling this way. Tell yourself that you feel this way for valid reasons — the baby you'd imagined is not the one you're having. It's normal to feel disappointed in this context, and more common than you think. Whenever you catch yourself feeling sad, disappointed, or frustrated, acknowledge this to yourself (e.g. 'I feel sad, as I was reminded just now that I wanted a baby girl').

Observing and naming what you feel in a non-judgemental and non-critical manner are key steps towards acceptance. Imagine making room for this feeling, breathing into it, and letting it be free to come and go. (Yes, this is easier said than done ... and this is where therapy may be helpful).

2. Reflect

Reflect on your preference. What does it mean to you have a boy or girl? Why is it important? Where does this preference come from? And what had you pictured regarding your ideal baby girl or boy?

When you're reflecting on this, it can be good to get these thoughts outside your head — discuss with a trusted person or write them down in a journal. Externalising your thoughts this way can help give perspective and clarity. And when you're taking perspective, consider the nature of your imaginings: how you imagined the baby girl or boy, and the things you'll do together are often quite stereotypical. For example: dreaming of getting your little girl dressed up, or seeing your boy perform at certain sports. And the hard part is that even if your baby was your idealised gender, they may not meet that fantasy, as they grow up to be their own person. You may never have gotten to watch your boy play footy — because he's a bookworm. Or you may never have gotten to dress your girl up — because she's a tomboy who wants to play in the mud. Consider that some of your gender disappointment may be due to a stereotyped gender image, and this image can drive some of your distress.

3. Mourn

The hard part is that we talk about gender disappointment, we are actually talking about grief and loss. You've lost the girl or boy that lived in your mind. And this is why it hurts — you're grieving your imagined baby and future. There are many types of loss, and not just from a death. When someone passes, there are rites of mourning to help you honour their life, their loss, and to say goodbye.

Grief needs to be felt and experienced, or it persists. If you are stuck in the loss of your imagined child, it can be helpful to find a way to farewell them and your imagined future. What sort of mourning can be undertaken to honour your imagined future? How can you say goodbye to the baby you'd pictured? It may not be as drastic as having a funeral or ceremony, but there may be small ways that you can acknowledge the loss you feel. Take time to think about what this might involve for you (it is often quite individual) and say your gentle farewell.

SECOND TRIMESTER

WEEK 14
Moving house when pregnant is no fun.

My thighs ached from climbing up and down the ladder to wash the ceilings. My nails looked like I'd been hand-digging graves in the backyard, so thick was the grime. Being pregnant excused me from lifting furniture and carrying boxes, but nobody thought I was too pregnant to help clean the house from top to bottom. At least my back pain had subsided.

We were moving out of an old Queenslander-style home with a big verandah and heritage cornices. It had plenty of charm and character, though some of the light fittings wouldn't have been out of place at an Addams Family garage sale. It was a cosy three-bedder and we were sad to be leaving. We'd found a new house to rent, located half an hour south of the city and much closer to my husband's work, which made sense given I'd be going on maternity leave soon.

My mother-in-law took on the tougher physical jobs like cleaning the oven, wiping down cupboards and mopping floors. This left me with the less strenuous — albeit still laborious — task of scrubbing every wall and ceiling. It was time-consuming, exhausting and involved more elbow grease than I'd anticipated. In the living room, I noted the slobber stains of Captain's jowl-shaking had somehow reached above the windows. *Why did I sign up for this?*

By 2pm I was FUMISED, but there was no way I wanted to come back and clean again the next day, so I pleaded with my body to keep going. I was so stiff every movement was like trying to ride my mountain bike uphill in the hardest gear. By the time we'd finished the entire house, my arms and legs were completely numb. Hobbling out to the car, I rebelliously chose to ignore a tiny black scuff mark on the front door jamb. I was done.

Husband and I collapsed on the couch in our new home that night and wearily glanced at each other. 'Next time we're paying someone to do this!' we said in unison.

For the rest of the weekend, I was forced to prop up my magazine against a cushion because I lacked the strength to hold it. I didn't move off the couch for two days.

BUMP BOX:
Ask for help!

The takeaway here is simple:

It's a good idea to get as much help as you can afford/unashamedly beg for, with any physical chores while you're pregnant. It might be something as small as carrying your groceries. If you're going for a long drive, you might want to consider asking someone else to get behind the wheel so you can stay comfortable. Perhaps get a friend to help you paint the nursery or move furniture around.

And in my experience, it's worth arranging someone else to help if you need to move house! Funnily enough, I know a lot of women who DID move house while they were preparing for their first baby ... and I can't recall any of them saying it was fun or great timing.

Nobody will shame you for asking for help, and it might just prevent an injury or free up energy that could be better utilised nurturing yourself.

WEEK 15
Welcome to Migraine City.

There it was again. An audible thud beating inside my brain.

I'd plopped myself in front of the television and surfed Foxtel, hoping for some air-conditioned entertainment during the heat of midday. I was pretty sure *Millionaire Matchmaker* was on around now. But the storyline wasn't really sinking in. It was so difficult to concentrate.

The last time I recalled having a headache was ... well, sometime before pregnancy and so long ago I really had no idea. It was probably on our honeymoon, the morning after the pool bar served complimentary half-litre plastic cups of cheap champagne. Before that day, I couldn't even remember having a headache, though I guessed I must have had them every now and then. Headaches weren't my thing. But headaches obviously didn't know that.

I wasn't stressed. I hadn't plied myself with happy juice and danced my bum off all night. My eyesight was fine ... So why the headache?

In my experience, while pregnancy doesn't allow for copious amounts of alcohol, it does allow for headaches of epic proportions and for no apparent reason other than the fact you're growing a human. But I never thought it would happen to me, since I'd hardly experienced so much as a hint of a headache before now.

The next morning it was back, eating away at my brain like a maggot on a rotten tomato. The headache put me off doing any useful work at the office, yet I didn't feel like it was a good enough excuse to ask to be sent home, so I just sat at my desk and went through the motions.

The following day, I had another obstetrician appointment, and I mentioned the headache, which had popped up again.

Dr McDelivery wasn't at all concerned. 'It's a totally normal, albeit annoying, part of pregnancy,' she said. 'All of your blood test results to date are excellent, and your blood pressure is healthy, so I wouldn't stress about it.'

We watched my baby wave and wriggle.

'At the medical imaging place last week, they said it was almost certainly a girl. What do you think?'

'I'd say a girl too. See these two white lines here?' My obstetrician pointed at the baby's downstairs bits. 'I'd say that's a vagina. If it's a boy, we can often see the scrotum instead.'

A girl. A beautiful, healthy baby girl. I was still getting used to the idea.

Not long afterwards, we were invited to my friend's little girl's first birthday party and something inside me permanently shifted. Watching Bethany and her daughter Elle together was so special. Elle was such a little lady, and the way Bethany spoke to her was so, well, feminine — for lack of a better word. It's hard to describe, but seeing two females together who share a bond is quite different to seeing a mum and her son together. The two females seemed to have an aura of gentleness and calmness, whereas I thought boys with their mums usually had more of a 'rough and tumble' vibe about them.

Both bonds were appealing, but I was starting to see why some people made such a big deal about baby girls. Having a girl. Someone who might actually enjoy watching rom-coms with me. Someone to go shopping with. Someone to ask me hair advice. Someone who will be on my team.

There goes that gender stereotyping again. Maybe my little girl will prefer horror films and want a crew cut. But either way, she will be awesome, right? She will be her own little person with her unique desires, dislikes and disposition. A baby girl. It had taken a few weeks, but my brain had made a definite 'switch'.

Around week 15 I had a solid boob-spurt. Not enough to make the cover of Maxim, but enough to force me to buy new underwear. I also started taking regular photos of my boobs because they'd never looked so good. I figured I'd want something to refer to once my child-bearing days invariably caused me to have saggy breasts; these photos would be a good reference for the future plastic surgeon who I hoped would be fixing my boobs.

These days, with phone cameras and filters, anyone would think taking a photo of your own chest would be a basic task.

But it just wasn't. I didn't even own a 'selfie stick'. It was a lot of trial and error, but after about 39 attempts, I managed to take the winning shot and proudly dubbed it a 'breastie'.

I pondered whether our national health insurance scheme, Medicare, should compensate all women wanting to fix their breasts after childbirth. As a country, we could change the first letter of our name and become BUSTralia. Because … tourism!

I wondered whether that was how BRAzil chose its name?

BUMP BOX:
Tips for taking the perfect 'breastie'.

1. Consider the angle. Are you using your left or right hand? Try to get your arm as straight as possible and face your phone camera as close to the middle of your chest as possible. (If you don't do this, one breast will look huge and the other will look tiny.)

2. Lighting isn't overly important if you plan to use filters. I preferred the yellow lights of my bathroom combined with the Vivid filter on my iPhone. Alternatively, get a spray tan.

3. Remember your posture. Don't be afraid to stick your chest out. I know it's hard to stand up straight when you have one arm extended at an awkward angle, but obviously good posture is essential.

4. Click the photo button on your phone. And voilà! You have a gorgeous breastie to look at and can reminisce for years to come.

WEEK 16
Finding time to spoil yourself.

Week 16 felt like week 116. I was like that sloth meme that reads: *I like to sleep a lot, so I have the energy to sleep more.*

I'd been led to believe the second trimester was often much better compared to the first in terms of energy, but it wasn't happening for me yet. I was so lethargic, I couldn't be bothered to do *anything.* Every day it seemed I was tired to the point where I felt ill.

I used to be up for sex all the time, but not anymore. I figured this must be what it was like for the first few months of being a parent — just too busy/tired for sex and too exhausted to care.

I wasn't exactly feeling sexy either, despite my bigger boobs. I was too tired to feel sexy. I stared despondently in the mirror at my widening hips and bigger bottom, my rounding belly, and thought back to my body just four months ago on our wedding day ... I no longer recognised any of these bits and pieces in the mirror.

I couldn't help but wonder while I was gaining a baby, was I also losing a part of myself? I wasn't looking like me, I wasn't acting like me, and sometimes I certainly wasn't feeling like me — where had the vivacious vixen gone?

Tired, unsexy, old me decided I should do something nice for myself to boost my self-esteem.

So, I made an appointment for a pregnancy massage.

'Lillian' was the perky girl I employed to make me feel great again. She was in her mid-20s with black hair and a lean frame. I'd been very clear on the Client Information Form — I prefer my massages very firm, and I was four months pregnant. Hopefully, despite being petite, she could really knead my muscles. Lillian asked a few of the usual questions: did we know the sex, had we picked a name, how long had my husband and I been together for, where did we honeymoon, etc. She told me about her son who was six and the father who wasn't around anymore. More power to her, I thought, for working hard to make a better life for her son.

There was so much chatter going on, I started to wonder when we were going to get to the 'massage' bit. Lillian had asked me to lie on my side, where she patted one half of my back as though she was holding a handful of jelly and trying not to spill it. Then she asked me to roll onto my other side ... by then I realised we were pretty much halfway through the massage.

What the?

I didn't want ask her to use more pressure at this late stage. And truth be told, I couldn't have asked her anyway ... Lillian hadn't stopped talking for the past 25 minutes.

'I've decided to take my son camping over the New Year; it's a privately-owned farm with ...'

'We don't have any computers in our house because he watches so much TV ...'

'He's such a smart kid and got this award in school the other day for ...'

'He was the first child to walk on the moon, and he once played the piano accordion on stage with Michael Jackson ...'

Okay, I *wished* she'd said that last one. My brain was shrivelling up in boredom. I reminded myself never to talk about my child this much after she was born.

One thing that did perk my ears up though was when Lillian told me she was 14 weeks pregnant before she found out. Yes — 14 weeks! I couldn't fathom not knowing that far along ... my body had undergone so many changes in those first few months it seemed crazy for someone not to realise. But then again, there are plenty of news stories about 'cryptic pregnancies', i.e. when women are unaware they're pregnant until they physically have the baby.

Between Lillian abusing my ears and the lack of pressure on my back, there was no relaxation to be had. *Shut up, please ...* So much for making myself feel better — a colonoscopy would have been more relaxing!

When it was over, I walked out the door and started to cry. I was just so damn tired and flat and forlorn, and nothing seemed to be helping. In saying that, I think a pregnancy massage — done right — would be a perfect indulgence for most expectant mothers needing a pick-me-up.

BUMP BOX:

I'm losing my identity, and baby's not even here yet!

The 'usual me' wasn't negative about my body, or negative in general. The 'me' I knew was full of motivation; I grabbed life and rolled around in a field of sunflowers ... *didn't I?* Not anymore. I hadn't even had my baby yet, and already I was a pile of procrastinating progesterone who became upset for reasons even I didn't understand. To be honest, I was scared. Would I feel like this forever? Was I the only pregnant woman on Earth who wasn't feeling empowered and positive and rainbows and roses?

This article extract from the Perinatal Anxiety and Depression Australia (PANDA) website (PANDA 2017) explained my feelings so well:

Loss and grief during pregnancy

Loss and grief are normal aspects of pregnancy, yet they are not often talked about. Holding a sense of loss and grief alongside the joy and anticipation of becoming a parent can feel confusing. Often expecting mums and dads feel shocked, guilty and ashamed by their feelings of grief and loss. So, they often push their feelings deep down inside.

Try to remember that it is common for expecting parents to feel the loss of a part of their sense of who they are, activities they enjoyed or their relationship with their partner. It can take some time to adjust to what they might have lost.

It can also take some time to really appreciate the new things they have gained. Some expecting parents feel ashamed by this unexpected grief, and if the feelings are not addressed it can impact their mental health and wellbeing.

Losses associated with expecting a baby

Here at PANDA we speak to many thousands of expecting mums and dads living with antenatal anxiety and depression. Many of our callers speak of loss and grief.

Here are some of the things expecting mums and dads tell us:

- *'I just don't feel like this is my body anymore'.*
- *'I'm worried that I might never get my career and level of income back.'*
- *'I really miss my mum. She died when I was young. I wish she was here to see me become a mum.'*
- *'My clothing doesn't fit anymore. And I can only wear pregnancy clothes, nothing that expresses my individual style!'*
- *'I don't feel attractive anymore.'*
- *'I miss not worrying about things I eat or drink. I miss having a drink!'*
- *'I've lost all my energy.'*
- *'I feel that I've lost my sense of possibility, of being able to have future plans, hopes and dreams.'*
- *'All that is in front of me now is this idea of becoming a parent.'*

This was so reassuring for me to read and hopefully will be for any of you who might be experiencing similar feelings. The fact organisations like PANDA even exist, says to me this is an area where many expecting mums need extra support.

WEEK 17
It's a Virgin Mary Christmas.

Spending the Christmas holidays pregnant kind of sucked. I know, I know, it's a small price to pay for the creation of life. But a usual Christmas for me involved a few glasses of champagne, gorging on glazed ham, wrestling with any children who popped by, and picking at leftover Boxing Day seafood.

So, to be honest, I was a smidge disappointed I couldn't do any of those things this year. And keeping with the theme of being honest, I did still enjoy the occasional wine during my pregnancy, though I'm not advocating anyone else should do the same.

Despite the obvious risks, pregnant women still drink alcohol for various reasons. Habit. Relief. Social inclusion. I drank a glass of low-alcohol wine every Friday throughout the second half of my pregnancy. (NOTE: I've read zero medical research saying low-alcohol wine is any safer; I just personally felt more comfortable drinking it.) The thought of completely abstaining did cross my mind, and obviously I was aware of the medical recommendations, but I felt okay with the amount I was consuming at the time. Drinking alcohol is a risk for every mum-to-be to consider, based on her own beliefs and values.

I have friends on both sides of the fence; some had a few glasses every now and then, others didn't touch a drop for the whole nine months. Nobody judged anyone else for their decision.

While in retrospect, I feel I probably should have quit the booze altogether (how horrified would I have felt should something have happened to my baby?), I was a bit sick of turning on the TV and having doctors and social commentators discussing and often condemning pregnant women for having even a sip of champagne on a special occasion. Now I was pregnant, it seemed as though every second program on television was about having a baby or raising a child and what I should and shouldn't be doing.

What next? Were people also going to make me feel guilty for having too much ice-cream and putting my baby at risk of being overweight? Were they going to tell me to stop crying because it might make my baby predisposed to depression? Were they going to tell me to stop rubbing my belly because I might give birth to a genie who wants to grant me three wishes?

Added to that, there was new information coming at us left, right and centre. For example, a study published by a researcher from the Reykjavik University in Iceland (James, 2020), concluded there was no safe level of caffeine for pregnant women — advising women to quit coffee altogether. The study reported results for one or more of six major categories of negative pregnancy outcomes: miscarriage, stillbirth, low birth weight and/or small for gestational age, preterm birth, childhood acute leukaemia, and childhood overweight and obesity. Caffeine-related increased risk was reported with moderate to high levels of consistency for all pregnancy outcomes except preterm birth. The study concluded 'current evidence does not support health advice that assumes "moderate" caffeine consumption during pregnancy is safe. On the contrary, the cumulative scientific evidence supports pregnant women and women contemplating pregnancy being advised to avoid caffeine.'

The inclusion of this study isn't intended to cause alarm — this is just one study and a summary at that — my point is I think you should make your own decisions based on awareness of potential risks and what feels right for you.

I often say about many life scenarios, 'There's no right or wrong; there are only different values.'

People will always speak and act according to their own belief systems and the knowledge they have, and that's what they will deem to be 'right' (even if I think it's wrong). I can't control what someone else finds right or wrong. I can provide information about my opinion and the reasons behind it, but I can't force anyone to agree with me. So, if a pregnant woman knows the risks behind something she's doing (slice of brie cheese, anyone?), I accept it's her body and her decision.

Not long after my merry-deprived Christmas, I grabbed my wallet and jumped in the car. Then I got back out of the car again to use the bathroom. Then I got back in the car, to go to the shops and return a few incorrectly sized/damaged gifts. Here's how the shopping trip went:

- Drive to shopping centre.
- Toilet stop.

- Go to Myer to swap men's t-shirts.
- Another toilet stop.
- Walk to bookstore to purchase book about how to make a baby sleep.
- Another toilet stop.
- Go to David Jones to swap cracked wine glass.
- Yet again, another toilet stop.
- Drive to service station to buy Husband a bag of ice.
- You guessed it! A toilet stop.

It was ridiculous. Pregnancy was making me soooo thirsty all the time, and all that water had to come out somewhere.

I decided all future shopping trips would be restricted to no more than three items, and I would only go to centres where I already knew the store layout and the most direct pathway to the nearest Ladies Room. And with any luck, my next pregnancy would be far away from the holiday season to ensure minimal shopping trips with an exploding bladder and maximum enjoyment over the holiday season.

BUMP BOX:

How safe is it to drink alcohol whilst pregnant?

The National Health and Medical Research Council website (National Health and Medical Research Council 2020) says pregnant women should avoid drinking alcohol altogether. Outlined in their 'Australian Guidelines to Reduce Health Risks from Drinking Alcohol' are several reasons behind this advice.

Women who are pregnant

Avoiding drinking alcohol during pregnancy prevents the risk of alcohol-related harm to the developing fetus. The existing evidence does not identify a safe amount of alcohol that pregnant women can drink. As there is a risk of lifelong harm to the unborn child, this guideline takes a precautionary approach and recommends not drinking alcohol when pregnant. The risk of harm to the fetus increases the more the mother drinks and the more frequently she drinks ... A variety of maternal and fetal factors can affect the risks from drinking alcohol while pregnant (e.g. genetic differences, metabolic rates, and biochemical and inflammatory responses to alcohol). These factors make it difficult to predict the level of risk in each individual pregnancy.

Source: National Health and Medical Research Council (representing the Commonwealth of Australia)

WEEK 18
Maternity un-fashion, the struggle is real.

'Oooh, I just love that maternity dress; I wish they made it in non-maternity!' That's something I've never heard anyone say, ever. That's because I've found most maternity clothes to be rather ugly, in particular maternity office wear. I decided to purchase clothes I would wear anyway, albeit in a larger size. That way I could either a) attempt to shrink them in the dryer afterwards, b) give them away to friends or family, or c) not bother losing the post-pregnancy weight so I could still wear them next season. In addition, I usually found buying regular clothes to be less expensive than buying specialist maternity-wear.

I went out in search of some maternity dresses to get me through the last few months of work, but I may as well have raided Ugly Betty's wardrobe. (Minus the fact hers was genuine couture.) All the maternity dresses I found that were 'work appropriate' for my conservative office were clashing-coloured, shapeless wrap dresses that made me look like I should have been wearing a badge saying, 'Hello! My name is Mildred.'

One maternity wardrobe tool I found very necessary was a 'waistband extender', which I used during the later stages of pregnancy. A waistband extender is a simple contraption consisting of a piece of elastic with a button on one end and a hole on the other, which can be used as a kind of 'belt' to join pants at the front in the zipper area, where they can no longer do up due to an expanding belly.

Waistband extenders saved me money; money that otherwise would have been spent on ugly work maternity pants. I found the waistband extenders most useful on shorts and work trousers. (For the record, I have never met a pair of elasticised maternity shorts that didn't look like a giant nappy.) It was also easy to hide the waistband extenders, as they can look quite messy, by wearing long tops to properly cover the waistbands.

All hail the waistband extender, fixer of shorts and pants, saver of money.

Please be wary of falling into the trap of buying too many maternity bras — now, some of these are quite pretty. But before you put your money on the counter, consider how far along you are, whether you're going to breastfeed, and if so, for how long. As a friend of mine put it, 'Don't forget that while you might be a C cup mid-pregnancy, by the time you reach 40 weeks, you could potentially be an E cup!' So, you probably don't want to be buying too many bras early on.

One other exception to the no-maternity-clothes-rule was some well-cut maternity jeans (I got mine at Top Shop), and they were the only maternity pieces I invested serious money in. I purchased four pairs and wore them to death. To summarise, I found it best to purchase minimal clothes during pregnancy and concentrate on buying accessories instead. Handbags and jewellery look good at every stage of pregnancy, and if you're fortunate enough to not get swollen feet, you can also spend your precious play money on shoes too.

BUMP BOX:

Are beauty treatments are safe during pregnancy?

While it can be challenging to find clothes that fit during pregnancy, you can still indulge in a little bit of fake tan and a mani/pedi, right? The RANZCOG website (RANZCOG 2020) explained it clearly:

Can you use fake tan during pregnancy?

The active ingredient in fake tan reacts with the cells in the outer most layer of skin, producing a brown pigment called melanoidin. Fortunately, it doesn't penetrate the skin much further, so isn't absorbed by the blood stream and therefore can't harm your baby. It's generally considered safe to use fake tan creams and lotions during pregnancy, but it's probably best to avoid spray tans, because the effects of inhaling the spray are not known.

Should you avoid manicures during pregnancy?

Just like hair dye, the chemicals used in nail treatments are in low doses and not readily absorbed by your skin. So, follow the same simple steps as for hair colouring to minimise potential absorption and therefore the risk to your baby.

If you have any cuts to the nail bed, its best to avoid any nail treatments and make sure your nail technician is using sterilised tools to prevent infections. If you don't know what kind of nail polish your salon uses, you need to advise them that they should avoid polishes that have dibutyl phthalate, toluene or formaldehyde in them. Fortunately in pregnancy, your nails are usually healthier and stronger, so for some women, manicures during pregnancy are not required.

WEEK 19
Doing the downward sprog.

I know this sounds ridiculous, but I was worried my baby would 'fall out of me' if I did any kind of high-impact exercise during pregnancy. This has never happened to anyone ever, but I always suspected I might be the first. Goodbye running and pump classes.

I decided to try pregnancy yoga instead. I'd attempted other types of yoga before and — TBH — not really enjoyed them. They made me feel anything but calm; I couldn't keep balance, and the poses required more flexibility than Bo Derek's bobby pins. However, I found pregnancy yoga simply delightful. *Easy* even. *Blissful.*

Our class started with a 20-minute meditation where our supermodel-esque teacher asked us to go to a series of 'happy places'. I went to the Lindt Factory and Eddie Murphy's house (my favourite comedian ever). Then we 'let go' of the issues that had been causing us anxiety all week. I let go of our neighbour's daughter's awful piano playing, which was a bit of a con really, because she was still playing when I got home. Regardless, the feeling was very nice while it lasted.

Our teacher then took us through an hour of stretches and poses, specifically designed to aid health problems that plague pregnant women. My favourite pose involved sitting on the ground and putting one foot over the opposite thigh then stretching forward, so I was lying forwards on the ground, but without my enormous belly touching the floor. This was an exercise we were told was helpful for insomnia (which I had A LOT of during pregnancy).

Then we did another stretch that was good for leg and foot cramps — boy, did I need that one! Twice this week I'd woken up in the middle of the night clutching my right calf in agony, and the pain seemed to transfer to my toes after a few minutes.

'Leg cramps are usually caused by a lack of magnesium,' the yoga teacher informed us. 'Dark leafy greens, nuts and seeds and dark chocolate all have lots of magnesium in them.'

The pregnancy yoga ended with us all lying on our backs, our legs resting vertically up the side of the wall.

'This will help more blood flow to the uterus to give your baby a rush of nutrients,' the teacher helpfully hummed.

I didn't understand exactly how that worked, but it sounded plausible.

While lying with our legs up the wall, we were encouraged to send loving messages to our babies and to continue breathing deeply. It was a nice feeling to take some dedicated time out to nourish my mind and body and concentrate on the fact I was having a baby. Life had been so busy, sometimes I forgot I was even pregnant.

To finalise the class, we did another meditation where we were told to lie on our sides with our eyes closed.

Which I did.

For a very long time.

Long enough for my girlfriend Soraya to go to the bathroom, pay the instructor, chat with some of the other girls in the room and for everyone else to leave. She finally gave me a gentle kick in the ribs and told me to wake up, which I was pretty dirty about because it was the best sleep I'd had in four months.

Husband and I watched a documentary once about the gruelling tests men had to go through to join the SAS in Australia. The men undertook punishing exercises day after day, with no sleep, to test their mettle. This was because sleep deprivation is a form of torture. I wondered whether sleep deprivation was a prerequisite to pregnancy, to ensure I was up to the task of raising a child.

There was the constant waking up because I had to pee, the struggle to get comfortable, in addition to the insomnia. I lay awake at night during most of my second trimester lamenting over the fact I had not yet purchased the necessary baby gear required to raise a child. I hadn't purchased a single thing; I hadn't bought a single singlet, bootie or teddy bear. It seemed like there was an overwhelming amount of stuff we needed, and I simply didn't know where to start.

At this stage, my baby would have nowhere to sleep, couldn't ride safely in our car, nor even be entertained with a single age-appropriate book. Thank goodness for the insomnia pose I learnt at yoga.

BUMP BOX:
What to look for in a baby bag.

There was one exception — the one thing I had ordered in preparation for the baby (though it hadn't yet arrived in the post) was a baby bag. The reason being, a friend of mine purchased no less than five nappy bags for her first baby — that's right, spent more than $1000 on these bags, before she found The One. She said none of her other baby bags compared to the 'style, convenience and practicality' of this bag, so I ordered one of the same.

I was fairly confident my friend was onto a good thing, given all of her experience.

This 'dream' bag contained pods inside — a temperature-controlled pod for baby food and bottles, a changing pod for nappies and creams, etc. — and it came with a built-in change mat, as well as a section for mums to keep their wallet and keys in. In my opinion, these are all very important elements. And it looked a bit fancy too.

It's worth doing your research on these before buying one, as there are so many options!

WEEK 20
Learn to take the good with the bad.

Was that the flutter of my baby moving? Or simply air moving through my intestines? I'd been paying more attention to my belly than I would an unsupervised bucket of KFC, yet I still wasn't sure if I'd felt a tiny human kick or if I was just hungry.

Now I was at the mid-point in my pregnancy, I was also finally starting to 'pop', that is, actually look pregnant. Well, I thought so anyway, but salespeople at the shops still looked confused as to whether to say anything to me.

'Popping' is a funny phenomenon. (Try saying 'funny phenomenon' three times fast — that's funny too.) I thought true popping occurred when your belly stuck out noticeably further than your boobs and started to look rounded. But again, what about those ladies who never even knew they were pregnant, and the baby just fell out one morning after a bowl of Special K? Maybe some people just never popped, I pondered.

At this point I was clocking between three to six hours sleep per night, broken up into several sections. So not only did I look like a crap kebab, I felt like I'd eaten it on a dirty street corner at 3am each morning. I wondered when my hair and nails were supposed to thicken, and my skin was supposed to glow ... isn't that what happens when you're pregnant?

Oh yes, sorry, I forgot. We're living in a time when it's all about positive body image and we're only supposed to talk about how 'strong' and 'functional' and 'womanly' our bodies are, right? I'm all for having self-confidence and thinking good things about myself; however, I was pregnant. I hadn't had any sleep, and I didn't feel empowered. I felt like ploughing my head into a cool bath of champagne-filled clouds, in a room overflowing with chocolate fondue. I wanted to whinge about whatever I wanted whenever I wanted, because that was my prerogative as a pregnant woman.

I was also starting to lose my centre of gravity. I was walking into door frames. I had trouble leaning forward to put shoes on, and I couldn't have been more uncoordinated if I'd strapped my belt around my ankles.

But a silver lining appeared, in the form of the frequency with which I had to shave my legs. It had decreased. Dramatically. Like, I'm talking going from shaving every second day to once a fortnight, and that wasn't because the weather was getting colder, and I could wear jeans. My leg hair just wasn't growing very fast at all. (Nor was my pubic hair, which was good, because waxing hurt a lot more when I was pregnant, which the beautician told me was because of all the extra blood rushing around my private bits. It's also worth noting here that I've had no less than 14 rounds of laser hair removal, and I still need to wax. I put it down to my Italian heritage — the hair follicles run STRONG on that side of the family.)

My bottom also looked very pregnant now. I'd never met a bum so hungry that it was eating up my full briefs, French knickers, Brazilian cuts and G-strings. It was getting big beyond uncomfortable. It was time to ... buy maternity undies, à la Bridget Jones. Alas, the wedgie-war was lost. I ended up buying undies at Bonds Maternity. But you know what? They were so comfortable, I felt like a total arse for not doing it sooner.

BUMP BOX:

Don't forget what you looked like before pregnancy.

I'd been taking weekly photos of myself from a side-on view so I could compare how big my belly was getting as time went on … for goodness sake, do yourself a favour and take at least one naked 'before' photo prior to becoming pregnant. Honestly, at 20 weeks, I looked at my 'four-weeks pregnant' photo and couldn't fathom ever having had a belly that small!

In saying that, also don't be in a hurry to get your belly back to what it was after giving birth. Bellies are not made of elastic, you know.

WEEK 21
What about PMS?

'Hasn't the dishwasher been unpacked yet?' asked Husband innocently. But in my mind, his tone was clearly stating, *'Why didn't you unpack it already?'*

WTF, I thought. *Turn around, numbskull. I've been unpacking the dishwasher for at least the last 17 seconds. You've been in the kitchen too, surely you can see me. Couldn't YOU have unpacked it earlier? Why are you asking this stupid question when you already know the answer? Now I will finish unpacking it before I have to pack it again with all the dishes we left in the sink this morning. Rather than standing there, judging, shouldn't you have noticed what I was doing and started helping me? Selfish pig. Stop looking in the fridge for dessert, or a glass of water, or whatever it is you're doing to stall for time and give me some help, moron!*

'No,' I replied, my jaw clenched. 'It hasn't.'

My husband has a few talents, one of which is that he's rather good at interpreting woman-speak. He immediately translated those three little words into, 'Please start unloading the cutlery tray right now otherwise I'm going to smash this Royal Doulton mug over your head.'

He kindly kicked me out of the kitchen, and I flopped onto the couch in a state of FUMIS.

I reflected on the interaction we'd just had and started to feel a bit guilty. I'd possibly mis-interpreted his tone. Perhaps I'd been a bit over-sensitive. Intuitively, I opened my period tracker app and noted that, had I not been pregnant, my period would have been due tomorrow.

Five whole months without my period. What bliss!

On the flip side, it became bleedingly apparent that while the physical signs of menstruation may have stopped during my pregnancy, the monthly hormone fluctuations hadn't. My earlier display of kitchen aggression proved I was still a short-tempered tyrant for a few days each month. During my period, I was tired, irritable, and short with people to the point where Husband would say, 'You've got your period, don't you?' and he was always damn well right, so I couldn't scream at him for the assumption.

'Sorry, honey!' I yelled in the direction of the kitchen. 'Have I been a bitch lately?'

'You've been pretty bad these past couple of days.'

'I just checked my period tracker app. Apparently even when you're pregnant you can still get the same hormone changes that cause PMS.'

'Ah, now your behaviour makes perfect sense.'

'Actually, I was chatting to your mum the other day and guess what? She said even after menopause, some women still get mood swings. She said it's possible to keep getting them for years and years afterwards. Maybe you'll be stuck with me being like this every month for the rest of our lives?'

'Uh-huh.'

Again, he had successfully translated my woman-speak into: 'I'm baiting you right now to see how much you really love me and if you'll put up with me being nasty to you once a month for the rest of our lives.' I gratefully accepted his concurrence as confirmation he would still love me ... though I'm not sure I would have been so forgiving if the situation was reversed: *'Listen Mands, I'm going to be a total a-hole to you for a few days ... every single month ... for the rest of our lives. But if you love me, you'll just put up with it, okay?'*

It wasn't just my 'mood' that was 'acting up' either.

I'd started to have sore boobs and initially wondered whether it might be related to PMS as well. There were sharp, stabbing pains in my left breast on and off all day, with no warning and nothing I could link to causing them. They persisted for several weeks, so I concluded it wasn't PMS-related. *What the heck is going on?*

Had someone created a voodoo doll and started pinching my boobs? The only way I found relief throughout the day was to sit at my desk, vigorously massaging my left breast with my right hand to try and ease the pain, while finger-typing press releases with my left hand. It was excruciating. (And simultaneously a wonderful source of entertainment for Clara.)

A quick check-in with several pregnancy forums on the internet reassured me this pain was most likely not, in fact, someone trying to spiritually assault me. Given I had no lumps or bruising, it was more likely to be just my expanding breasts adjusting to growing milk ducts. I made a note to check with my doctor, just to be sure.

Did you know women have an average of nine milk ducts opening onto the nipple in each breast (Ramsay et al, via Australian Breastfeeding Association 2021)? Up until my pregnancy research, I had honestly thought it was just one big, fat round milk duct in each boob. Was I a complete idiot? Did every other woman on Earth, except for me, know this? I couldn't believe I didn't understand the biological make-up of my two closest companions, so I wondered how I was ever going to figure out breastfeeding.

Breastfeeding was a bit of a contentious issue for me, given I had inverted nipples – Stage Three inverted — meaning the nipple is impossible to pull out for any length of time. (Once I had an operation that was meant to bring them out, but they ended up popping straight back in again, so it was a rather brief meeting.) The nipples still exist, they're just inside of my breasts so you can't see them. Where a nipple would normally appear, instead is a small indent in the areola about three millimetres in diameter.

And no, I'm not the only one. I've known a woman who had one inverted nipple whereas the other protruded normally. I once knew a girl who could pop both of hers in and out with her fingers. Plenty of women have them; it's a thing.

It was a topic of endless discussion when I was at high school. I regularly got asked about them by my classmates, for example, 'What do they look like? Can you put coins in them?' and 'Have you tried putting ice on there?'

Well, I've tried just about everything to coax them out. I even tried to suck them out with a vacuum cleaner when I was 16, but all I got for my troubles was a boob hickey. I was really hoping to breastfeed my baby, but I didn't have high hopes due to the severity of my inverted nipples.

Many of my friends who already had babies had said breastfeeding wasn't easy. Some of them didn't enjoy it. Some of them loved it. I'd accepted my inverted nipples were going to be an additional hurdle. And, truth be told, I was trying not to think about it because it was that time of the month again and I didn't want another reason to feel anxious.

BUMP BOX:
What is PMS?

For this definition, I looked to Australia's first and largest specialist hospital dedicated to improving the health of all women and newborns, The Royal Women's Hospital. Their website (The Women's 2020) explained premenstrual syndrome clearly.

Premenstrual conditions

It is common for women to experience physical changes as well as changes in their mood a week or so before their period starts each month. These changes are called premenstrual syndrome (PMS) or premenstrual tension (PMT).

PMS can include:
- *irritability, moodiness, impulsiveness, anxiety and/or feeling a 'loss of control'*
- *a depressed or lower mood*
- *difficulty concentrating*
- *bloating, swollen and tender breasts, and body aches.*

These changes can be mild, moderate or severe. They can last for a day or two, or right up until when your period arrives. Some women only have physical symptoms, others only mental ones and some women a mix of both.

PMS can be so strong that it can affect your ability to do the things you normally do.

WEEK 22
A natural remedy for congestion.

Josie and I had been friends since the first year of high school. She's one of those super smart people who can look at just about any problem and automatically know the answer because 'It just makes sense, doesn't it?'

Despite having rarely lived in the same time zone for more than five minutes because she travels so much with her job, we've kept in close contact over the past couple of decades. Josie gives terrific advice, and she's loads of fun to be around — two major attributes I look for in a life-long friend.

Josie and her husband had not long completed yet another international relocation, this time to London, when I got a Skype call.

'I just vomited on myself. During peak hour on the tube.'

'OMG. What did you do?'

'What was I supposed to do?' she said. 'If I got off at the next stop, it wouldn't really achieve anything, as there are no bathrooms at most tube stations, so I just sat there and kept riding until I got to where I was going. I'm sure the other passengers were mortified.'

'What are you going to do now?'

'Go to work, I guess.'

In true, professional-Josie style, she went to work, cleaned herself up and got on with her day. It was one of the few bad decisions she's ever made ...

Less than two hours later, she leaned over a colleague's shoulder to discuss some work and threw up again, simultaneously destroying a keyboard, a notebook and the girl's expensive blow-dry.

Josie worked for a major global company you would have heard of (and by 'worked', I mean she oversees thousands of people across several continents in a number of different time zones, so I can't even begin to understand her definition of 'work'). While I was pregnant and 'settled down', she and her husband were living the high life with a fabulous apartment in central London, where they still went clubbing on weekends, and she had time to make sophisticated cocktails. They'd been married for more than a decade and children were not on their agenda, anytime soon. Josie had suffered from endometriosis since she was 16 and used the Pill to keep the pain under control; the thought of not being able to take the Pill was terrifying because her endo was so terribly painful.

Several more spew sessions later and you guessed it ...

'I'm pregnant!'

'Congratulations! This is awesome; our babies are going to be close in age!'

Given her chronic endometriosis and the fact she was using birth control, it had never occurred to Josie she could possibly get pregnant.

The Endometriosis Australia website says it's estimated more than 11 per cent of Australian women or those that identify as gender diverse will suffer from endometriosis at some point in their lives, and that up to one third may have difficulty becoming pregnant.

Josie felt that being pregnant was a miracle of the finest order. Josie's good news was just the pick-me-up I needed, being in the midst of a nasty cold. Coming down with a cold when you're pregnant is the absolute pits. Husband drove me to the chemist on the very first day to 'knock it on the head', but all that achieved was me wanting to knock the pharmacist on the head.

'I can only advise you to take some Panadol and get some rest,' he said.

ARGH! I felt my burning throat and stuffy nose were far beyond the powers of Panadol.

Four days later, I was twice as congested and doubly fatigued, so I went to the doctor.

'I can only advise you to take some Panadol and get some rest,' she said. 'And I'll give you a medical certificate for a week off work.'

The following day, I developed post-nasal drip; the constant stream of phlegm between my nose and my throat, which made it hard to swallow. The symptoms kept coming. Watering eyes. Brain fog. I felt just awful.

A week away from the office was nice, but I was desperate to get better. There's only so much time you can take off work before you start feeling guilty.

ENTER THE 'NETI-POT'.

While it sounds like something used in marijuana farming, this unusual contraption is a natural remedy for congestion and post-nasal drip. I won't lie to you, using a neti-pot is not a trip down to Fun Town. But I was pregnant and sick and desperate for clear sinuses and didn't have a lot of other options.

The woman at the health food shop handed it to me; it

looked like a miniature teapot. The instructions said to mix one cup of lukewarm water and a quarter teaspoon of salt into it. On the advice of the naturopath, I bought some stupidly expensive Himalayan salt (apparently pouring in a heap of Saxa cooking salt isn't the same thing). Anyway, once I had the salt and water mixed inside the neti-pot, the instructions said to stick the spout of the teapot into one nostril and tilt my head forward at an angle so the water flowed into one nostril and came out through the other nostril. (Obviously, I did this over a sink.) Then, once I'd drained half of the pot, I repeated the process, tipping the water into the other nostril first.

Remember when you were a kid and your friends would take you by surprise and dunk your head under in the pool and all the water would go up your nose? It felt like that. But I got used to it, and the results meant I could breathe and swallow more comfortably for a few hours.

I used it twice a day for three days and it improved my post-nasal drip significantly; I'd recommend one for a bit of congestion-relief. But I was still feeling fatigued; there was no way I felt well enough for any kind of physical activity. And my brain was still foggy.

So, off to the doctors I went ... again ... and received a subsequent antibiotics prescription — which was something I'd hoped to avoid, but as it turned out, I'd developed a severe sinus infection.

'Amoxycillin is what we call a Category A antibiotic,' the doctor assured me. 'It's considered safe for pregnant women to take, and I think you're going to find you'll need an antibiotic to get over this nasty infection.'

Watching television, reading and sleeping were fun activities, but doing them for weeks on end was starting to affect my mental health. So, I took the antibiotics and was back at work in three days.

I held onto the neti-pot though, which turned out to be a good decision. This may have been my first ever sinus infection, but it wasn't my last.

BUMP BOX:
What is endometriosis?

The Endometriosis Australia website (Endometriosis Australia 2021) says the condition is caused when tissue similar to the lining of the uterus is found outside of the uterus in sites around the body (usually in the pelvis), but it has been found as far away as the brain.

Endometriosis Australia says it's important to understand that while the current evidence suggests that women with endometriosis are more likely to experience fertility problems, not all women with endometriosis will need assistance, and only a small number of women will require IVF.

According to the organisation, the only way to diagnose endometriosis with 100 per cent certainty is to see an Endometriosis Specialist Gynaecologist for the appropriate tests, namely a laparoscopy (a thin telescope is placed into the belly button), with a biopsy (tissue sample taken) for pathology testing.

WEEK 23
Is that my baby kicking?

It happened so quickly I could barely fathom it. One day I was happily tucking my pregger-tummy rolls down into the waistband of my jeans; the next day the jeans were so tight I couldn't have squeezed a bee's penis down there. I jumped on the scales at week 23 to discover I'd suddenly gained an extra 3.5 kilograms.

By now, strangers were asking 'How far along are you?' and my mid-section was starting to get double takes in the street. To top it off, someone almost sat on me at a local rugby match, presumably mistaking me for an overstuffed couch.

Everywhere I looked I saw other pregnant women. It was like a highly contagious disease spreading throughout my regular haunts ... restaurants, the local shopping centre, the nature reserve where I walked Captain; they were all filled with pregnant women now. Or had they always been there, and I just didn't notice them?

I found myself purposely touching my belly in public ALL THE TIME. This was to inform staring strangers that *yes, I know you're just checking as to whether I'm pregnant before you comment. Yes, see, I'm touching my belly!*

People had begun to offer their seats to me at our

overcrowded work meetings, and for the first time in my life, catching public transport wasn't such a bad thing.

Up until now, it had been easy to forget a lot of the time that I was growing human life inside me; however, all of that was about to change ...

Husband and I were watching *The Wolf of Wall Street* at the movies. There was an awful lot of swearing in the film (in fact, the f-word is used more than 500 times) and plenty of arguing between Jordon Belfort (Leonardo DiCaprio) and his wife Naomi Lapaglia (Margot Robbie). During a particularly loud and aggressive scene, I grabbed Husband's hand and whacked it on my stomach. Our baby was reacting to the heated cuss words blasting through the speakers!

'I felt it!' Husband yelled, in a voice slightly too loud for a cinema.

'So, I'm not imagining things?'

'No way, that baby is kicking hard.'

We grinned and shared one of those fuzzy, electric looks.

I spent the following days trying to find a 'pattern' to my baby's (non-induced) kicking, as instructed by the midwives on the internet. Several websites had said I should keep a record of this 'pattern', so I'd know what was normal/abnormal for my baby's movements — this way I'd hopefully be alerted if there was something wrong.

From around 2pm until dinnertime was when our baby was kicking the most, but I wondered whether that was just because

I generally tended to be busier at work in the mornings, so I wasn't consciously feeling her kick then. In addition, with my placenta sitting on the front of my uterus acting as an additional 'barrier' (as opposed to being positioned on top or to one side), it was hard work for me to feel any kicks that weren't super strong. I did my best to be conscious of the kicks, but I can't say I felt as though there was any distinctive pattern for me, personally.

Now that my baby bump was rather large and moving around, and so very real, I felt 'properly pregnant' — for lack of a better expression. For me, being 'properly pregnant' meant my centre of gravity was confused, and my coordination skills were edging dangerously towards extinction. My tiredness had peaked through the roof, making my clumsiness worse. I was permanently FUMISED. I had 'Baby Brain'. I was repeating myself; yes, I realise how repetitive I sound right now as I complain about these things. Bottom line was, much of the time, I felt exhausted and useless.

Well, I guess I wasn't exactly useless ... anyone need an overstuffed couch to sit on?

BUMP BOX:

Tips to feel your baby move.

After that first instance of our baby kicking, I wanted to feel it all the time. Some of my pregnant girlfriends had tried and tested this method:

1. Lie on your left side.
2. Drink a cold glass of juice.
3. Feel your baby kick.

While I can't find any medical evidence to support this 'tip' (i.e. please don't take it as a fail-proof method), it worked for me! I believe it's something to do with the coldness of the liquid and the sugar in the juice encouraging the baby to move. IMPORTANT: if you're ever concerned about the movements of your baby while in utero, always consult a medical professional for proper assessment.

WEEK 24
Too many veins and not enough sleep.

Anytime we happen to be lost, my friends ask me which way to go and then choose the opposite route, which invariably gets us to the desired destination. However, suffering from orientation-deficit was no longer a problem now I was pregnant. Help was at hand. Literally. I had developed a road map — in the form of bulging veins — on the backs of my hands. Who knew a hand had so many veins? All I needed to do was pick one and write 'You Are Here' at the bottom, and I would probably get commissions from the Tourist Information Bureau.

My hands looked like they belonged to a 90-year-old. I couldn't comprehend how this weird-vein condition related to pregnancy; I'd never heard anyone talk about how freaky their hands looked while they grew a baby.

The road maps weren't just restricted to my hands either. My bum could have been used for a game of Snakes and Ladders, and what I found fascinating about my veiny bum was the number of women I spoke to who'd had a similar experience. It's not an exact figure, but a survey of my child-bearing circle of friends would put the figure at about 99.89999 per cent. Despite this staggering statistic, veiny hands and bums while pregnant was something I'd never heard about before; I felt there really should be some kind of Public Service Announcement explaining this weird phenomenon.

At 24 weeks, our obstetrician told Husband and I our baby was now 'viable'. This basically meant it had developed enough to be born with a chance of survival (though a very, very small chance at this early stage). She said around 50 per cent of babies born between 23 and 32 weeks survived, though obviously most of those were closer to 32 weeks.

This information provided a small amount of comfort in my constant sea of worry. There was hardly a day that went by I wasn't worried my daughter's heart had stopped beating or I was going to go into early labour. Then I couldn't help but think of all the potential things that might not go as we planned, even if the delivery was fine. Our baby could be born with developmental difficulties, she could roll off the change table when I wasn't looking, or what if I got carjacked while she was in the back and someone drove off with her? I guessed all the worry was just part of the whole motherhood preparation thing; weren't mothers constantly worrying about everything?

Seeing our baby kick around on screen in the obstetrician's office was always a joy. It was well worth the 45-minutes-to-an-hour-and-a-half spent waiting (it seemed like there was always a baby born unexpectedly on our appointment days). Each appointment only lasted about ten minutes, which included the ultrasound, the consultation and the weigh-in. I wished our appointments were longer; to see more of our baby and discuss every thought/scenario/concern that had gone through my head since our last appointment — or since time began — and get our doctor's opinion on every single thing. Then I read somewhere: *a short obstetrician's appointment is a good thing, as it means there is nothing wrong,* which made me feel better.

It was around this stage of my pregnancy I started to inhale the contents of my fridge and pantry every five minutes. My stomach never felt full. Eating the equivalent of a small supermarket every day felt unavoidable. To paint a picture for you, pre-pregnancy, a typical day for me used to go like this:

Breakfast: ½ cup of porridge with skim milk and a teaspoon of sugar.

Second Breakfast: Ham and low-fat cheese toasted sandwich on wholegrain bread.

Lunch: Leftovers from dinner the night before (this could be anything from spaghetti bolognese to a roast dinner).

Afternoon Snack: Small freddo frog.

Dinner: Whatever my husband cooked — lamb and salad wraps, salmon with steamed vegetables, chicken curry, etc.

Now my days looked more like this:

Breakfast: ½ cup of porridge with skim milk and a teaspoon of sugar, followed by a thick Italian dark hot chocolate on the way to work.

Second Breakfast: Ham and low-fat cheese toasted sandwich on wholegrain bread, followed by whatever leftovers I was originally planning to eat for my lunch.

Lunch: Having already eaten my lunch before lunchtime, I'd be forced into the city streets where I'd try to find something pregnant women were *allowed* to eat … and there was nothing I 'felt like' … which is why most days I'd end up buying a bag of soft, white bread rolls and a tub of butter.

Afternoon Snack: Small freddo frog. Thankfully I always had the foresight to keep a supply in my top drawer at the office. But this was no longer enough to keep those afternoon sugar cravings at bay, so sometimes I'd leave the office again for a chocolate gelato thickshake.

Dinner: Whatever my husband cooked me. This was generally followed by me saying, 'Baaaabe ... I'm still so *hungry*. Would you please go buy me some ice-cream?'

To which he would reply, 'I asked if you wanted me to buy you some when we did the grocery shopping on the weekend, and you said no.'

And I would say, 'Yes, but that's because I was trying to be healthy. I want to stay healthy for you and *for the sake of our baby*. But to be honest, it's really the baby that wants ice-cream. You can't tell a baby it can't have ice-cream, *it won't understand*.'

'It's almost 8pm, I don't really want to go to the shops, honey. I'll get you some tomorrow.'

'But there's nothing else in the house I — the baby — *wants to eat*. And it's so *hungry*. We both are. *Pleeeease*.'

And because my husband knows from experience the only way to shut me up when I'm complaining is to either feed me or have sex with me, he'd mentally debate which was the more attractive route from his point of view and head in that general direction.

I knew this food trajectory couldn't continue, and I certainly wouldn't recommend this diet for anyone else – but I honestly felt very hungry and was simply eating what I craved.

Baby steps, I told myself. I made a pact to cut out the Freddo from then on.

The constant peeing was becoming unbearable. I was waking up at least five times a night to use the bathroom and then had a huge amount of trouble going back to sleep.

My doctor said pregnancy insomnia was sometimes caused by anxiety. *Pffft*, I internally scoffed. *Me? Anxious?* I was only a bit worried about something going wrong before or after the baby was born and slightly concerned about being underprepared for the whole thing. But surely I wasn't anxious, was I? I then stayed awake most of the night wondering whether I was anxious, which of course answered my question.

I was considering asking to cut back my work hours. An extra two hours at home would make a big difference to how early I could get to bed and how much more sleep I could potentially get, particularly with this insomnia keeping me awake so much. But the thought of asking my boss to let me cut back my hours gave me heart palpitations and made me sweat, so I decided not to say anything, plus I didn't want my pregnancy to result in extra work for my colleagues.

I wished there was some sort of map or guidebook to help me navigate these sorts of conundrums, but not even the back of my hand was providing any direction.

BUMP BOX:
Should I be eating for two?

The RANZCOG website (RANZCOG 2020) explains:

Many women are unaware of how much weight they should put on during pregnancy and some gain more than is ideal. A pregnant woman only needs to add a portion of extra calories to support her baby. The exact quantity of calories depends on your weight, height, level of activity, whether or not you are overweight, as well as the trimester of pregnancy.

Pregnant women should be advised to eat a healthy, well-balanced diet and on an average, consume about 350–450 additional calories per day during pregnancy (the equivalent of two healthy snacks such as a piece of fruit, hard-boiled egg, hummus with vegetable sticks or berry smoothie). There is no need to 'eat for two' as was previously thought.

WEEK 25
Men don't always listen.

Pregnancy is like a construction site. There's so much hardcore activity going on — loosening joints in your body like someone's taking them apart with a screwdriver, your heavy load creating new muscles, the spreading of hormones like wet concrete, cells multiplying at the rate of a dropped box of nails. I was growing another brain inside of me, while my own brain chucked a sickie ... for example, I mistakenly threw $20 into the garbage bin one morning, because it was sitting next to an empty milk bottle on the kitchen bench. Then when I went to the shop, of course I had no money to buy milk.

Popping into the shops was now proving difficult. I felt like there was a cement slab always strapped to my belly. My arms and legs moved in slow motion as though they were trying to break free from superglue. My headaches were like a nail gun to my skull. There were times I felt I'd swallowed a jackhammer — but it was most likely my intestines and stomach adjusting to make room for the baby. My sweet child's legs were constantly poking me in the ribs, and I had concerns she might kick hard enough for an outright demolition.

As Husband and I walked through a housing estate one day, inspecting new constructions, Captain was running into puddles, sniffing trees, and bounding up to other dogs we met along the way.

Husband pointed out a large concrete house slab with the frame established. 'That's a massive house,' he said. 'None of that stuff was even there when I walked past the other day; they haven't mucked around putting it up.'

'Look at all those pretty colourful parrots sitting nearby,' I replied. 'There are hundreds of them.'

'This one looks like it will be the first — no other houses look even close to being started yet,' said Husband.

'I can't believe how many parrots there are; don't you think they're cool? Captain, I bet you'd love to chase those parrots through the field, but they'd fly away before you could get within ten feet.'

'I guess it makes sense since none of the frames are built by hand anymore; they're all manufactured in a factory.'

'I wonder where they all sleep at night. I've never seen them around here before. Is it breeding season? Honey? Do you think it is? Babe?'

The sound of parrots screeching.

I'm sure he would've thought the parrots were nice to look at, if he'd take the time to listen to me. *Why are you not listening? Is this not the most intriguing question I've asked today? Perhaps of all time? WHAT ABOUT THE FACT THAT THEY ARE GREEN AND RED WITH A BIT OF YELLOW?*

A rational, non-pregnant woman would realise it was okay for a man not to give a rat's kahuna about a pretty bird. (And to be totally fair, Husband started speaking first.) But I'm blaming pregnancy for losing my previously sound mind. It was almost like I was having an outer-body experience. My body and mind were no longer my own. Men must understand that if a

116

pregnant woman says the old lady licking the feral cat carcass is pretty, then they must STOP, LISTEN, and AGREE. I was building the equivalent of a show home. I deserved respect. *Sigh.* There were days when Husband had the emotional intelligence of a deaf newt on crack.

'Honey, look! The parrots are drinking out of the pond!' I exclaimed.

'I think they're going to build a second floor,' he replied.

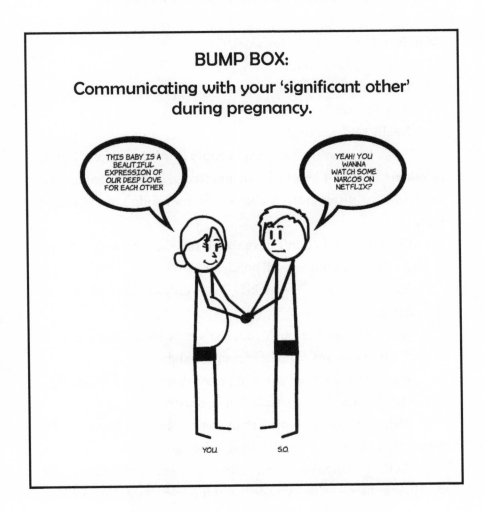

WEEK 26
What about antenatal classes?

'Mandy, what do you do for work?'

'I'm a media advisor.'

'Oh, really, that must be exciting! Who do you work for?'

'A politician.'

'Really? Which one?'

'Ah ... I generally don't say. People think I can fix all their problems if I do.' I laughed half-heartedly. Telling people who I worked for often started conversations I didn't want to get into.

'Of course. You don't have to tell me.' *Long silence.* 'So, is it [insert name of controversial politician]?'

'Umm ...' *Eye roll* — luckily, I was only speaking to her on the phone.

'Sorry, I shouldn't push you. Let's move on. Have you ever in your life taken any kind of recreational drug?'

'Well ... yes ... I tried smoking marijuana at high school.'

'I see.' *Disapproving hum.* 'Only once?'

'Well, probably more than once, but I don't really remember. School was such a long time ago.'

'Well, I suppose I can leave out the part about the marijuana then — since you only did it a few times. Yes, I guess that would be okay.' *Sound of pen taking notes.* 'What about STDs, have you ever had any of those?'

'I'm sorry? Could you repeat the question?' (Are STDs pills or powder? I pondered.)

'STDs — Sexually Transmitted Diseases. Have you ever had one?'

'Oh! STDs! No, I haven't.'

'Have you ever suffered from depression, or anxiety?'

'Well, we all get anxious from time to time. But no, I've never been clinically diagnosed with either of those things.'

'What about Husband? How is he coping? Is he cool, calm and collected?'

'Usually, yes. He's a pretty calm guy, except for when he loses his temper, obviously.'

'Oh, really? Interesting. Does he lose his temper often?'

'No, not really.'

'Are you sure? You can confide in me safely.'

'He really doesn't.'

'Does he hit you?'

'No!'

'Has he ever threatened you?'

'Absolutely not.'

'Mandy, are you concerned he may be violent towards you in the future?'

'NO! He is a wonderful man. *Everyone* gets angry. I probably frighten him more when I lose my temper, than me vice versa. He isn't violent at all!'

'I see. Hmmm. But he does get quite angry? Does he verbally abuse you?'

'Well, not really. I mean — no, of course not!'

'Okaaay ... hmmm.' *Sound of pen ticking boxes.* 'Have you

decided how you plan to feed this baby?'

'Well, I'd like to breastfeed. However, I do have inverted nipples, so from what I understand it may be a bit more challenging for me.'

'Oh, of course you can breastfeed. Good. And as for your inverted nipples, you just pry them out with your hands. Breast is best, dear.'

'Well, mine are Stage Three inverted. I've had an operation to try and rectify them, but my nipples only appeared for a short period of time then disappeared again. You can't just bring mine out manually, like pulling a coin out of a wallet or something.'

'An operation? Really? Tell me about your operation.'

'It was just a minor operation, where the doctor basically put a barbell through my areola, like a piecing, to try and stretch the nipple to come outside of my breast. As I said, they stayed visible for a while after the piercings were removed, but then they disappeared back inside again.'

'That sounds rather painful.' *More pen ticking.* 'Did it hurt?'

'What do you think? Why don't you ask someone to shove something the size of a biro through your boob and see how you like it? Come on, are all these questions seriously on your list or are you just a nosey parker? And for goodness sake, stop making judgmental noises with that fucking pen!'

Okay, I may not have answered that last question in exactly that way, but *if* I could have been 100 per cent certain the midwife on the other end of the phone was also not going to be in the delivery room with clear access to my vagina and newborn baby, I honestly can't say how that conversation would have ended.

To me, my hospital 'pre-admission phone interview' had felt more like courtroom cross-examination. Some pre-admission interviews are done in-person, which I think in my case would have felt more comfortable, given the level of personal information they were asking for.

Trying to cover my inappropriate giggles, I was watching a woman well past her child-bearing years sitting on a stool with her legs apart, holding a resin pelvis on her lap and pushing a plastic baby in and out of it. It was pretty weird to watch. The woman then held a fake breast up to her chest while a plastic baby 'sucked' on it. I knew I was being immature, but there were more than a couple of muffled laughs from 'classmates' in all corners of my antenatal class who were obviously feeling a similar level of discomfort.

In fairness to the presenter though, how else was she supposed to teach the class about giving birth?

Anyway, the one-day intensive class went from 9am until 5pm. I found it disconcerting the teacher didn't take her handbag off THE ENTIRE TIME. Did she leave it over her shoulder in case the class suddenly broke out in riotous laughter at her fake baby-birthing and she needed to make a quick getaway?

Overall, though, I found the class to be very enlightening (Husband tuned out for most of it). I especially enjoyed learning about the 'Three Stages of Labour'. Honestly, before this class, I thought the 'Three Stages of Labour' were:

One: Your waters broke. **Two:** You went to hospital, and; **Three:** You pushed your baby out.

As it turns out, giving birth is quite a bit more involved than that. Here's what I learnt in class about The Three Stages of Labour.

Stage One

This is when your water usually breaks, and your cervix starts to dilate. The definition of 'Stage One Labour' is when your contractions start to become regular, e.g. 20 minutes apart for a while, then 15 minutes apart for the next while, etc.

During early Stage One, you're only dilated up to three centimetres. Your contractions are usually mild, and apparently if you're in bed when this starts, you can even go back to sleep. (*Really? Who goes to sleep when they're about to have a baby?*)

As Stage One progresses, your contractions start to become more intense and last for about one minute to 90 seconds at a time, every three to four minutes. (This is when most women are told to hightail it to the hospital.)

The presenter told us that by the end of Stage One, we'd be ten centimetres dilated, we'd probably be feeling exhausted, and the contractions would get closer together.

Stage Two

By Stage Two, your cervix is ten centimetres dilated, with an urge to push. This is when the 'climax' occurs. (Not that kind of climax — though I did read online that some women do orgasm while they're giving birth.)

The climax is when you need to start pushing the baby out of that ten-centimetre hole. By this stage, contractions are back to every four or five minutes apart, as that way you can push during your contractions and have a rest for a few minutes afterwards. But hey, you don't really need to remember any of this stuff because hopefully there'll be a midwife and/or an obstetrician there telling you exactly what to do. (That is, unless you don't make it to the hospital in time and must give birth en route. One guy from my high school graduating year delivered his own child because his wife's labour was so short — so it does happen!) This is the stage where you should see the baby crown, then one baby shoulder pops out, quickly followed by the other shoulder, then the rest of the body just sliiiides through. (Obviously not everyone's baby is delivered with the ease of a greased-up contortionist, but this is how it's ideally supposed to go.)

Though most won't, babies can get stuck. This might lead to one or many different interventions: forceps, an episiotomy, a doctor's hand as well as a baby inside your vagina, emergency caesarean, etc.

Stage Three

But you haven't finished yet. Mother Nature twists the knife in harder and you find out you have to deliver the placenta too, because growing and pushing out a little human wasn't challenging enough. While some women are so enamoured with holding their baby at this point that they barely even notice pushing out their placenta, others may find this to be an additional, unexpected hurdle.

Anyway, once the placenta is out, then you're all done making a baby; the chaos of parenthood ensues.

Alternatively, if you happen to have a planned caesarean, this can potentially be a much more straight-forward process than outlined above. But one way or another, your baby will come out into this crazy wide world, and you will be a Mama. Welcome to Parenthood!

The antenatal class also taught expectant mothers to let their partner/anyone else in the room at the time, change the first nappy. To demonstrate why, the midwife held up a chart displaying photos of different types of baby poop.

The first dirty nappy your baby creates will usually contain about 20 WEEKS WORTH OF POOP. This poop mound has just been hanging tight inside your baby for months. It's thick, black and looks like a terrible makeup accident involving too much mascara and a bit of green eyeshadow.

The class also covered how to swaddle a baby, and they gave us a tour of the hospital. (The hospital tour was the only part Husband was interested in.) The presenter showed us where to park the car when we arrived, which desk to check in at, and where the birthing suites and maternity ward were. I hadn't spent a lot of time in hospitals before; they smelt funny. I supposed that's why people always sent flowers.

There was also a physiotherapy part of our antenatal class, run by a sweet girl called Mary. The best part of this class was when Husband had to give me a massage, rubbing two tennis balls up and down my spine for five entire minutes, which was four and a half minutes longer than any massage he'd ever given me at home.

Mary explained why people should always give pregnant ladies their seat on the train and not let them lift heavy things; I'd previously thought this was because pregnant ladies were huge, tired and angry. However, it's because a hormone called 'relaxin' loosens pregnant ladies' joints a lot, therefore any sudden or unusual movement might cause serious physical damage.

Everyday activities I took for granted, such as pushing a grocery trolley or lifting a stack of magazines, could cause me to pull a muscle or put a shoulder out, thanks to relaxin. Relaxin was also responsible for loosening up the pelvis joints, which would help make my pelvis big enough to fit a baby through — I'd always wondered how something so relatively large, like a baby, could fit through something that was also designed to fit a penis in snugly. It was the ol' pelvis-widening hormone trick. Again, this is a good reminder to take all the help you need during your pregnancy, even with the small tasks.

The biggest lesson I took home from the physio class was that I'd been getting into bed the 'wrong' way. Rather than just clambering in via any means I could manage, I should have sat on the edge of the bed, then lay down sideways, then rolled over onto my back and gotten comfy. Getting in and out of bed willy-nilly can (and did for me) cause strain and/or injury. I now knew why I'd noticed sharp pains in my belly when I 'forced' myself into bed in a careless fashion.

Mary also explained how to properly sit for long periods of time, such as at a desk or in a car, saying it was best to have a small pillow or rolled up towel behind the lower back to prevent slouching/spine strain.

Finally, the other very important lesson I learnt was that my pooping style was totally wrong. To lessen the risk of haemorrhoids (um ... what?!), Mary said 'number twos' should always be undertaken sitting on the toilet seat, leaning slightly forward, with my feet on a little stool. This position would help to straighten out my colon, meaning the poo could sliiiiide right out — as opposed to having to navigate a bend.

(Trying to be helpful, I explained the correct pooping position to colleagues at the office the next day and they looked at me like I had just told them the Earth was round. Was I the only person on the planet who didn't know how to poop correctly?!)

'But if you take one thing away from tonight,' concluded Mary, 'it's to brace as often as possible. Everyone sit up straight and tighten the pelvic muscles, just like you would if you were to stop peeing mid-flow. Now hold it. Feel how firm your core is during this position. This is bracing. I want you to do three sets of ten, three times a day. And definitely brace when sneezing and coughing. Does anyone know why we do this?'

I think all the females in the room knew, but no one wanted to say the word.

'Incontinence,' Mary filled the silence. 'After you have a baby, your pelvic floor can become weak. We need to strengthen it as much as possible beforehand, so you can control your bladder. Partners, husbands, what are you going to say every time your partner sneezes?'

Again, silence.

Husband helpfully chimed in with 'Come on!' thinking no one could hear his whisper, but the room was so quiet, he may as well have been yelling. You could feel the other men in the room silently questioning whether his horse had come in.

'Did you BRACE?' Mary answered, covering the awkward atmosphere in the room.

126

Part of me wanted to shove the tennis balls into a place ... hmm ... the other part of me figured I'd bide my time and make him wear a t-shirt covered in placenta blood. You read that correctly, I'd recently discovered from various friends that you can *do* things with your placenta!

BUMP BOX:

Fun things to do with your placenta.

Save your placenta and get creative with some of these interesting activities.

Make it into jewellery. There are a surprising number of businesses online that use either the placenta or umbilical cord, jazz them up with resin, and make them into bespoke pendants and beads. Gift for the new grandmother, perhaps?

Create art. You can use the blood from the placenta to create a beautiful piece of abstract art. Hang it in your child's room and wait until they're a teenager to tell them how it was created, so you can be certain it will totally gross them out.

Paint t-shirts with the placenta blood. Matching Halloween costumes, anybody? (Albeit somewhat unhygienic, I imagine ...)

Plant it. Some women feel like the placenta was such an important part of their baby's life, they want it to 'live on' — so they put it in the ground and plant a tree on top.

Encapsulate your placenta in pills and swallow them. Did you know you can purchase DIY Placenta Encapsulation Kits? The

---

kits enable you to grind your placenta into powder form, put it into a capsule and swallow them one at a time. Potential benefits to these pills might include more balanced hormones, enhanced milk supply, and lessening the severity of any postpartum depression. There are also professional businesses that specialise in completing this process for you, as cleanliness and precision are important in encapsulation.

There are plenty of other placenta activity suggestions available online, if this is the sort of thing that floats your boat.

WEEK 27
Why is everything suddenly blurry?

Laser eye surgery was one of the best things I've ever done. (Having my eyes lasered, that is — not doing it to somebody else of course. I'm not that clever.) My experience entailed four large, sharp pieces of metal clamping each eye open for around an hour. Eye drops were popped in to numb my eyeballs, then I'd watch the little tools come towards me ... closer ... closer ... boom. Scalpel in, laser pointed, eyesight changed.

By the next day, I was able to see clearly for the first time in years. It was like turning the lights on for the first time. Like a microbiologist inspecting fungus, I took so much pleasure in just LOOKING at stuff. I'd had no idea the tops of my feet had light, fluffy tufts of hair on each one. Imagine what else I had missed!

I'd worn glasses since I was eleven years old, initially just to read the blackboard at school and for watching television, but as the years went on, I became more and more short-sighted.

For example, when playing touch football, I couldn't see the ball from the other side of the field. As I walked through school, I'd return the gesture of someone waving hello, only to find as we walked towards each other that I had no idea who the person was (and they were, embarrassingly, waving to the person walking behind me).

At 14, I decided to get contact lenses, but they only worked out well for a couple of years. Once I started drinking alcohol and going to parties, contacts were too high maintenance. If I forgot to take them out, they'd end up stuck to my eyeballs like Blu-tac on an old NSYNC poster, often followed by some kind of eye infection. These infections prevented me from wearing my contacts for the rest of the week, therefore defeating the purpose of having contact lenses in the first place. So, by the age of 19, I'd saved up and paid the price to see clearly again through laser eye surgery.

And in the 14 years since then, I'd never had a single problem with my eyesight — until week 27 of my pregnancy.

First off, my right eye started feeling 'furry'. Far-away things I used to see clearly, such as street signs and people, became blurry. And there was a nagging pressure constantly pushing behind this eye. So, I tried to figure it out.

Day after day, night after night, I'd repeat eye exercises using different targets. For example, I'd cover one eye and read letter-by-letter the small text on a brochure stuck to the wall at the other end of the office. Or I'd cover the other eye and see how clear people's facial expressions on the television were. After doing these exercises for a couple of weeks, it was clear to me (or not clear, as was the case) there was something wrong with my right eye, and it had nothing to do with how much sleep I wasn't getting, or what time of the day it was.

Was it something to do with my eye operation all those years ago?

The female optometrist looked down at my belly. 'Oh, you're pregnant? And you can't see properly? Totally normal, my dear! I'll take a quick look at it but come back and see me if you're still struggling with your sight when your baby is six months old.'

Excuse me?

'Quite often the eyesight will just go right back to normal once your hormones settle down,' the optometrist said. 'I wouldn't worry too much, your sight is still very good, even though I realise it may not seem that way when you're comparing one eye to the other.'

She then did the standard eye check to confirm her suspicions and sent me on my way.

Those pregnancy hormones sure had a lot to answer for. I was bloated, uncoordinated, irrational, anxious, bladder-capacity compromised, FUMISED, and now I was half-blind. It was a reasonable analogy for this whole pregnancy thing really; I felt half-blind to so many things I thought I should already know. How could I have the best pregnancy if I was so damn clueless?

BUMP BOX:

Why can pregnancy blur your vision?

Optometry Australia's 'Good vision for life' website (Koh 2020) helped me see things a little more clearly. It states:

Pregnancy hormones fluctuate constantly in a number of different ways, and more-often-than-not these hormones make your body produce fewer tears, thus causing dry eyes.

In stark contrast to this, some pregnant women retain fluids, and the side effects change the thickness and shape of their cornea. Women who suffer from this experience distorted vision; however, the condition usually goes away after they have the baby.

For others, interrupted sleep and hormonal changes that continue to play a part in the early months of having a newborn baby may continue to cause dry eye symptoms.

Thankfully, in my case, the distorted vision did settle down within a few weeks of giving birth.

THIRD TRIMESTER

WEEK 28
What's the blood glucose test?

I'm one of those people who needs to eat breakfast immediately upon waking otherwise I go a little crazy. Ever seen one of those wildlife shows where a pride of hungry lions fights over a recently deceased carcass? That's me without my Weet-Bix.

Being pregnant compounded this tenfold.

Today, however, I wasn't allowed to eat until 10.30am when my blood glucose test would be finished. The blood glucose test or 'the Pregnancy Oral Glucose Tolerance Test' is a routine blood test for pregnant ladies that ascertains whether you may or may not have gestational diabetes.

The test itself was not unpleasant. Upon arrival, the lone worker at the Pathology Clinic asked me to drink some very sweet cordial. That was fine.

Half an hour later, he drew blood from my right arm. Then half an hour after that, he drew blood from my left, then my right arm again another half hour later. The resulting bruises were on the large side. But that was fine too.

What sent me into abysmal despair was that the test went for two and a half hours, yet there were no magazines, no radio, no television, no newspapers, no pamphlets, absolutely nothing in the waiting room. These were the days well before COVID-

19, so I didn't think my expectations were unreasonable.

Phone scrolling on social media only killed so much time. I played 'I Spy' with myself, but the only things in the room were three red plastic chairs and a poster about the Red Cross, so I just ended up giggling at the ludicrousness of the situation and how bored I was.

At this point, I'd been in the waiting room for only 20 minutes.

The plastic chair put my back at an awkward angle, which made my belly uncomfortable, and the air-conditioning was blasting down into the waiting room at a ridiculous 18 degrees, according to the wall gauge. Given it was at least 26 degrees outside, I hadn't thought I'd need a jacket that day.

'Do you mind if I go next door to buy a magazine?' I enquired politely to my 'blood extractor'. The newsagent was literally at the bottom of the staircase leading to pathology, one shop to the left.

'No, you can't,' he grunted back. 'Some women react badly to the sugar drink and can pass out, so for liability reasons you must stay put within physical sight of the office at all times.'

Based on his tone, I suspected Pathology Man was sick and tired of being asked this question. Or he hated his job. Or both.

'I'll be back in less than two minutes, and if I'm not, I promise not to sue,' I pleaded.

'You can't go,' he replied robotically, and I noticed a sweat patch under his arm. Eww.

'How can you not have any magazines in here? And couldn't you turn up the temperature in this room?' The effects of my non-existent breakfasts was starting to come into play.

'It's not that cold in here, is it?' he replied, obviously not really caring either way.

'Are you kidding me? I'd rather be sitting in Hell when it freezes over. That room where you drew my blood isn't half as cold as the waiting room — and you get to sit in there where it's nice and warm (*and obviously you sweat your butt off*), but I'm expected to sit out here in the freezing cold for two hours? Can I at least sit outside in the corridor? It's a glass door, so you'll be able to see me.'

'You want to sit outside the office? There's no air-conditioning out there.'

'Exactly my point!'

I dare say happily, he picked up one of the hard, plastic chairs and put it outside for me. About 45 minutes later, a woman came by the pathology office carrying patient files. She kindly enquired if I was there for the blood glucose test.

'Yes, how could you tell?'

'It's very cold inside that office, isn't it? My patients say that a lot. I don't blame you for being out here. My office is right down the hall, I'll bring you back some magazines shortly.'

The Pregnancy Gods really do exist.

About 15 minutes after that, a male doctor came by.

'Are you in the naughty corner?' he joked.

'No, I just have to be here for two hours and it's like the North Pole in that waiting room,' I said with a wry grin.

He gave me a kind look and went inside, returning a moment later with my 'chipper' blood extractor, who told me it was time to come in for my next needle.

'You really should turn the temperature up in that waiting room,' the doctor said to him. 'It's too cold for her in there.'

'It's not cold in there!' he protested.

'Yes, it is.' The doctor made it sound so matter-of-fact. And no Pathology Man could argue with a doctor — rank successfully pulled. I gave the Doc a silent high-five and gigantic smile. After he walked away, Pathology Man turned the temperature up three degrees!

Today would change future conditions for all pregnant women who walked into that pathology office for their blood glucose test. I decided if my uncomfortable two and a half hours made the world a better place for them, it had all been worth it.

BUMP BOX:

Tell me more about gestational diabetes.

According to the RANZCOG website, gestational diabetes is a form of diabetes that occurs during pregnancy and usually goes away after baby is born (RANZCOG 2019). Gestational diabetes is common, with more than 35,000 women being diagnosed with the condition or its recurrence each year in Australia, and 3000 – 4000 women in New Zealand. Extracts from the website read as follows:

Certain factors increase a woman's risk of developing the condition.

Who is at increased risk?
Moderate risk factors include:
- *Ethnicity: Asian, Indian Subcontinent, Aboriginal, Torres Strait Islander, Pacific Islander, Maori, Middle Eastern, non white African*
- *Women who are above the healthy weight range.*

High risk factors include:
- *gestational diabetes in a previous pregnancy*

- *previously elevated blood glucose levels*
- *age 40 or over*
- *family history of diabetes or a mother/sister who has had gestational diabetes*
- *previous large baby with birth weight above 4500g*
- *polycystic ovarian syndrome*
- *some drugs or medication.*

How is it diagnosed?

Gestational diabetes does not cause obvious signs or symptoms in most pregnant women. It is usually diagnosed during routine screening performed at 26 – 28 weeks of pregnancy. The Pregnancy Oral Glucose Tolerance Test (POGTT) is used to assess how your body responds to a glucose load.

Why does it need to be treated?

Gestational diabetes that is not carefully managed can result in high blood glucose levels, which may cause problems for you and your baby. Keeping blood glucose levels in the normal range, reduces the risk of complications and increases the likelihood of a straightforward pregnancy and birth.

WEEK 29
Buying the essentials ... what *are* the essentials?

'I just need your help to buy three things, honey,' I implored. 'I know how much you hate shopping, but let's just go and buy the pram, the cot and the baby car seat. You'll be the one putting them together, plus you'll need to know how to use them anyway.'

This was woman-speak for: *the pram, the cot and the baby car seat will be entirely your responsibility. I'm not technically minded enough to assemble them, and let's face it — if I try and fail, I'll get stressed out and take it out on you. So, come shopping with me and let's avoid the possibility of both of us having a crappy day.*

We strolled into the baby store and spent about 20 minutes browsing around and saying things like 'Ahh' and 'Yes, that looks nice' and 'Hmmm' before realising neither of us had any idea what we were looking at.

'Can I help you?' enquired the sales lady.

I've just spent five minutes studying how to hang this mobile above a cot we don't have yet, before discovering it was a breast pump attachment. Yes, you can help me.

'We're looking for three things: a pram, a cot and a baby car seat. Both of these car seats look fine; what's the difference

139

between them?' I asked.

'They're just different year models of the same seat. That brand is about the best on the market.' She proceeded to show us all the shock-absorbing bits and other safety functions of both models, how each could be adjusted as the baby grew, how the seat faced both backwards (when they are young) and frontwards (as they got older).

'How do you wash the seat after the baby gets food and vomit on it?' asked Husband, in a manner that nearly convinced me he knew how to use a washing machine.

The sales lady demonstrated how different sections of the car seat fabric were attached together with clips and straps, but I was immediately confused. The sections were awkwardly shaped and stretched over so many different parts of the seat, I was sure I'd never remember the process.

'Getting the bits and pieces off to wash them shouldn't be too much of a problem,' I said to Husband with a grimace. 'It will be getting the pieces all back on again in the right places.'

This was woman-speak for: *every time I wash this car seat, it would be great if you could take all the bits of fabric off and put them back on for me.*

The seat we chose (last year's model, since as far as I could tell the only differences were the available colours and the price) came in a colour called 'praline', which we chose due to its similarity to baby vomit colour therefore less likely to show stains.

Telepathically high-fiving each other for making that decision relatively quickly, Husband and I moved onto prams.

'It only takes a jiff,' said the sales lady as she picked up a three-wheeled model. 'You just push these white buttons, grab the two red levers, move them left and right, remove the handle by untwisting this bit here, hold the pram by this long part and this short part and move them inwards — that's step one of folding. Then you simply unscrew this thing and stick your arm in here, pulling it towards you and folding it like that. Finally, unclick these ones, tuck them into the sides, rotate the wheels to the left and make this section fold here, and then you'll be right to pop it into your car boot.'

Uh-huh.

It seemed like all the prams had a convoluted process for setting up, pulling apart and folding. They each had so many optional attachments, such as raincoats, drink holders and shade cover clips, that they should really have had their own dedicated store. We walked from one end of the shop to the other, looking at all sorts of prams and getting more and more confused about the right one for us.

Various friends had given me a heads up on some popular brands, but what I hadn't realised was there were about a million different models of each brand. If I liked the look of one, I didn't like the tyres. If it had the right tyres, Husband didn't think the suspension was good enough. If we both liked the style of one, neither of us liked the colour selection. I really didn't know if I preferred three wheels or four. What difference did that make anyway? We both wanted a pram that had the option of converting into a two-seater, in case our second baby came along quickly.

I'd finally narrowed it down to two, when Husband walked over to the other side of the shop, pushed a black-and-rainbow-coloured pram under my face and said, 'Mandy, look at the butterfly print on this one. Our little girl would love this.'

'Do we really need to spend that much on a pram?' Seriously, my first car had cost less.

'Look — it's only three steps to fold down. And it looks awesome. It's perfect.'

The ease of functionality combined with my tough, tradie husband going gaga over an Andy Warhol butterfly print was enough to sell me. As was the fact we'd been looking at prams for more than an hour and a half, so I just wanted to pick one. A quick test to ensure it fit into the boot of my hatchback, and we were sold. Added to that, the sales lady offered us a $250 gift voucher to the store, which made me think we'd gotten a decent deal on the pram after all. It didn't convert into a double pram, but by this point in the process, I don't think we'd have minded if it turned into a pumpkin at midnight, we just wanted to decide on one.

Next up, the cot. I'd seen a gorgeous one online that converted from a cot, into a bed, into a table and chair set, but it failed to impress me when I saw it in person. It just didn't seem very sturdy. There were cots that converted into double beds, cots with matching change tables, cots with adjustable height functionality, white cots, birch cots, antique-coloured cots, dark-brown cots, and cots so secure they could have doubled as a tiger enclosure at the zoo.

As we walked the perimeter of the store several times going through all the different room displays and having the sales expert explain the pros and cons of each cot, the time we'd spent at the store started catching up with me. I suddenly felt extremely thirsty and tired. This was obviously not unusual, as there was a little corner with a couch, magazines and a water cooler for moments like these.

I collapsed while Husband grabbed me a drink and we pointed to various cots from our nesting spot. We decided on a white cot with matching drawers and a change topper, then went to the counter to pay for our exciting new purchases.

'Oh, I'm sorry,' the sales lady said. 'That cot is out of stock for the next 12 weeks.'

Husband and I looked at each other, knowing our baby was due in ten weeks, but neither of us could fathom having to spend one second longer looking at cots or anything else to do with babies. Our heads hurt, our feet hurt, and I was dangerously close to being FUMISED. We'd planned to borrow a Moses Basket (this is a portable sleeping basket, for small babies, that you can pick up and walk around with if necessary), so that would have to do while we waited for the cot to arrive. We paid and filled in the necessary paperwork.

'I guess you're driving home, babe,' I said.

That was woman-speak for: *I can't possibly cope with any more thinking baby or doing baby at this moment, and now your exhausted wife is going to have a nap in the car before her head explodes and her baby brain splatters all over the new baby car seat, and for crying out loud, I just can't baby anymore and just drive the freaking car already please so I can sleep and pretend I am not in fact babying at all.*

While the shopping trip had been a success, I felt like there was still so much to learn. I'd heard of a bassinet, but still had no idea what one was. How was it different to a Moses Basket? Does a breast pump require special batteries? Exactly how necessary was an automatic nappy bin? How many nappies will I need in the first week? What should I take with me to the hospital?

BUMP BOX:

It's okay to buy second-hand.

Don't you just love the smell of new furniture? Me too. I bought everything brand-spanking-new for my first child, but in hindsight there were a few things I wish I'd saved money on. Babies are EXPENSIVE.

This idea was first brought to my attention when a relative showed me the cot she'd purchased off Gumtree for her first child, and I literally couldn't tell, no matter how closely I looked, that this item had been used before. All that had been purchased was a new mattress. The cot was gorgeous and cost less than half the price she'd have paid for it brand new.

Fact is: small babies don't always wreck things.

To give you an example, we did a lot of travelling when our daughter was a toddler, so we bought a small travel pram. We paid hundreds of dollars for it — more than I thought we should for a secondary pram, but it was light to carry, sturdy to use and easy to fold. After about 15 trips away, it was still in great condition, but we didn't need it anymore, so we gave it to a friend who ended up using it as her primary pram for her child.

Another example is playpens — in my opinion, these are not an essential item but may be handy in certain situations. I didn't use one, but a quick hunt online showed me there are plenty available online, almost new, at heavily discounted prices. It's worth doing a bit of research if you're counting your pennies. Importantly, ensure anything bought second-hand meets the requisite safety standards.

WEEK 30
The truth behind big, black granny undies.

My heart raced and my face contorted into zombie-spotting fear when I heard the news. One of my colleagues, Sharona, had given birth to her baby on Wednesday ... and she'd only started her maternity leave on the FRIDAY PRIOR. Her precious little girl had arrived three weeks early.

Wha?

This possibility hadn't even occurred to me. Just last week, Sharona had said to me she'd been having nightmares about being one of those women who finished work and then had their babies almost straight away — something to do with your body finally relaxing properly, so the baby therefore thinks that it means it's time for them to 'arrive'.

Evidently, this was a real thing.

A thing I did *not* want to be a part of.

That cannot happen to me, I told my baby. I needed 'me time' in between work finishing up and the baby arriving. I had solid plans for those five weeks of 'mat leave', namely:

- moving house (yes ... again)
- getting a Brazilian
- learning to meditate
- purchasing the rest of the required baby paraphernalia

- watching the US season of *The Bachelor*
- and catching up with friends who I probably wouldn't see much of in the first few months following the birth.

I sternly informed my unborn baby that her early arrival would mean:

- she'd be parting thick coils of steel wire hair with her bald scalp during the birth
- we'd have nowhere to live
- she'd have nothing to wear.

However, in case my daughter turned out to be the rebellious kind, I thought I'd best start packing my hospital bag. I popped in some maternity pads, each the size of one of my Havaiana thongs, because a lot of bleeding can happen following childbirth. To cater for these enormous pads, I also packed several pairs of gigantic black undies, the belly button-reaching type that completely covered my ample bottom.

This in turn reminded me I wanted to groom in preparation.

I'd never given Russell Brand my phone number, so I concluded he wasn't hiding down my pants, I just really needed a wax. I borrowed Husband's hair clippers to give myself a 'number one' in preparation for my visit to the beautician for a Brazilian. But it didn't seem to matter how I stood or sat, or where I put my legs, I just couldn't see what I was doing due to my enormous belly.

Not to worry, the plastic comb on top of the blades pretty much guarantees I won't cut myself, right?

Somehow ... nope.

My lady parts were haemorrhaging like a bloody sprinkler. *Why didn't I use a mirror? Good question, you idiot.*

A mirror came in handy the following day, to see if there

were any signs of visible scarring or scabbing following my hack job.

There were no cuts.

There were no scars.

It looked as tidy as the neighbour's cat's bum.

My vagina was relatively normal looking ... if you don't mind a bad 80s haircut.

But ... yep, there they were — haemorrhoids. They looked like what I can only describe as three small leprechaun fingers trying to claw their way out of my bottom. It took all my self-control not to throw the mirror on the ground and scream.

I was so confused. I'd done all the things the physiotherapist had recommended in the antenatal classes to prevent them. I'd leant forward to do a bowel movement, never strained. I'd eaten plenty of fibre. What if these pesky, purple pods were mortifyingly multiplying?

I was lucky they weren't painful or itchy, as I'd been told haemorrhoids could be. I wondered how long they'd been there for.

I'd heard haemorrhoids described as 'varicose veins of the anal passage', which I interpreted as 'swollen blood vessels around the bum hole'.

They are nothing to be ashamed of — many pregnant women get them. I know because I asked them. *I'm not ashamed. I just want the leprechaun to have his freedom. Free the leprechaun. Ariel, my love, please free the leprechaun.*

Online forums I read were divided between women whose haemorrhoids had gone away on their own two to three months after delivery, to those whose still hadn't gone away 12 months on, and then those who'd needed surgery to have them removed many years later. These women touted warm baths, ice packs and lashings of witch hazel on the bulging veins to remedy them, but just as many said they hadn't had any success whatsoever trying to ease the symptoms.

I added some witch hazel to my hospital bag, then pointed my bare bottom in the direction of our swearing jar, in hope this pot of gold might entice my little leprechaun to climb out.

Nope.

Thankfully, my OB had a Plan B.

BUMP BOX:

What should I pack in my hospital bag?

I researched on the internet, asked friends, and gave it a great deal of thought: What do I take to the hospital? What are the necessities, and what little luxuries will make my visit more comfortable? Here's what I came up with.

My hospital bag list:
- Obstetrician's contact details
- Medicare/Private Health Insurance cards
- Paw paw ointment
- Phone charger
- Pineapple juice (I'd been craving this all pregnancy.)
- Spare clothes/underwear/shoes and swimmers — apparently you can take long, hot showers during the labour, if you want/if time allows
- Bathroom essentials, i.e. toothbrush, toothpaste, shampoo, conditioner, moisturiser
- Makeup and nice clothes to wear home (The midwives

will sometimes insist on taking photos 'of this momentous occasion' as you leave the hospital with your first child.)

- 10 x pairs of big, black cheap Bridget-Jones-style undies
- Pyjamas (ones that button all the way down the front are a good idea if you want to breast-feed)
- 6 x packs maternity pads
- Nursing pads
- Nursing bras
- My own pillow
- Books/magazines (NB. These turned out to be unnecessary, as I didn't have time to read a single thing post-birth. I was too busy attending breastfeeding classes, seeing physios, nurses, doctors, trying to breastfeed, trying to sleep, seeing visitors, etc.)

For HUSBAND: spare clothes, underwear, shoes and boardshorts.

For THE BABY: Nappies, wipes, singlets, clothes. (It's a good idea to check what your hospital provides so you don't pack too much — some hospitals provide nappies and wipes.)

WEEK 31
Rogue 'rhoids are to be expected.

'Oh, they're very common, I have just the stuff.'

My obstetrician wrote in capital letters on a post-it: PROCTOSEDYL. 'Just take that to the pharmacy. You can also try ice. At the hospitals we fill condoms with ice and use those for haemorrhoids.'

And we use those condoms like an icepack, I assume ... I hope.

Waddling through the city with wriggling leaches in my pants was the easy bit — handing over the post-it note in a subtle manner at the pharmacy was far trickier. I artfully used my hand to conceal the word written in CAPITAL LETTERS from those in the queue behind me just in case someone knew what PROCTOSEDYL was.

'Oh, I'm glad your doctor's gone straight to this; it's the best stuff. My sister-in-law got REALLY BAD HAEMORRHOIDS with all her kids!' exclaimed the pharmacy assistant, embarrassing my entire being so much that I'm sure my engorged little veins were desperately trying to escape via the nearby dark hole.

I swallowed my indignity and accepted the tube with a grateful smile, hoping with all hopes I was carrying a cure in my hands. *There's no way I'm rubbing this on my bottom at work,* I thought, *it'll have to wait until I get home.*

Veins, veins, veins. While haemorrhoids were never on the list of something I thought I'd have to endure, varicose veins were a different story ... When I was 12 years old, I was getting schooled up by DOLLY Doctor in a waiting room, while my mum was seeing the real doctor to 'have her veins done'. Mum's twisted, swollen veins had appeared on her legs during pregnancy and never gone away. Mum's veins had bulged out of her legs to the point where she was often in pain when she walked. I remember her doctor telling me varicose veins were hereditary, so I should be vigilant about drying my legs in the direction of my heart after a shower to try and prevent them from occurring.

Anyway, this particular day, Mum was wearing pants (as opposed to a dress) and these particular pants had elasticised bits around the ankles, which would have been the fashion back then. She was also wearing new shoes, brown and green leather flats with pointy toes; I remember thinking I would have liked some in my size. But regardless of a shoe's street cred, they lose all appeal when they overflow with blood, and said blood sploshes all over the waiting room carpet.

It took a while for people to notice. Mum was paying her veins bill, oblivious to the growing red puddle at her feet. But then she slipped as she turned away from the counter, and a wave of confusion washed over her face, followed by a downward glance and a choked voice. 'I'm bleeding!' yelled Mum.

'Doctor Barnes!' yelled the receptionist.

'Your shoes!' I exclaimed.

The doctor came straight back out and whisked Mum away again, assuring me everything was going to be fine.

Thankfully, the river of blood was nothing too serious.

Prior to her surgery, Mum had rolled up the leg of her pants to give the doctor access to her veins. However, this meant the elasticised bottom of the pants had effectively acted like a tourniquet, stopping the blood flow. After the surgery and the rolling down of the pants' leg, there was a torrent of blood that burst her stitches. The stitches were easily mended, but Mum's new shoes were ruined.

Being young and impressionable, I thought varicose veins were something I wanted to avoid at all costs, and so far, I had.

An old school friend, Simone, who shared the same due date as me, hadn't been so lucky.

'Varicose veins are like someone has punched me in the leg and it really hurts!' she complained. 'I don't know what to do about them. And then there's the stretch marks ...'

'Gosh, don't even talk to me about stretch marks,' I replied. 'You should see mine! But they're not from being pregnant, they're from when I lived in London.'

There were faded lines all over my body, permanent scars from when I lived in the UK and gained 15 kilograms in just a year and a half. Despite the fact I wasn't eating loads of junk and was still going to the gym three times a week, the weight simply attached itself to me like a colossal squid trying to hitch a ride with a whale. (This specific type of rapid weight gain for foreigners in the UK is famously known as 'The Heathrow Injection'.)

During my overseas jaunt, I outgrew nearly my entire wardrobe approximately every three months. And though I can't complain about the forced shopping, the necessity of owning clothes that legitimately covered my body in the freezing temperatures completely decimated my bank account. In fact, I returned to Australia with a $3000 credit card debt and a relative who told me I'd grown 'fat in the face'. *Lovely.*

The weight gain had caused bright purple stretch marks on all my curvy bits, top and bottom. Then upon moving back to sunny Australia, the weight mysteriously disappeared as though it had evaporated. But by that stage, my skin had already done some serious stretching; an extra 15 kilograms on my frame was fairly substantial.

Five years later, the stretch marks were still there, albeit a little faded — shiny lines snaking across my breasts, my hips and my thighs, patterning my skin like tally marks.

My belief (hope?) was that if I gained less than 15 kilograms during pregnancy, then surely the stretch marks couldn't get any worse?

BUMP BOX:
Can stretch marks be prevented?

If you're experiencing stretch marks, you're not alone. But they may be here to stay. Dermatologist Cathy Reid, Fellow of the Australasian College of Dermatologists, says stretch marks are very common, particularly during periods of rapid growth spurts such as pregnancy.

'I'm not aware of any cure for stretch marks,' she said. 'The good thing is, when you're pregnant, they may appear livid and purple, but in time they will fade to a silvery colour. I'm not aware of anything that can prevent them either — a lot of people use things like Vitamin E cream or Bio-Oil, and while these are safe to use, they aren't guaranteed to be a magic fix.'

WEEK 32
Is baby's hair to blame for my heartburn?

Simone and I continued to chat (well, complain to each other) throughout the following week.

'The heartburn! It's awful, Mands. It feels like a hot pain rising through my body,' she said. 'I've tried using a probiotic, and I've even cut back further on coffee — which you know is a big deal for me — but if it keeps up like this, I might have to go to the pharmacy to get an antacid.'

Simone said heartburn happened when the pregnancy hormones relaxed the valve separating the oesophagus from the stomach, and acid was regurgitated … but I'd heard pregnancy heartburn was because your baby had lots of hair.

Was it one, the other, or both?

Heartburn was a common complaint among my pregnant friends, who had tried to remedy the symptoms with anything from eating avocado to using extra pillows, with a mishmash of results. The upshot was that different things worked for different friends. (Of course, if you're experiencing persistent heartburn, please see a medical professional for advice.)

Simone and I also discussed waters breaking. One of my girlfriends (who shall remain nameless) had taken herself to hospital a couple of years earlier, thinking her waters had broken. She was extremely upset — waters breaking at her early stage of pregnancy could have been fatal for the baby. The medical staff hooked her up to all the machines and did an internal examination to try and find out what was going on.

Fortunately for her, her 'waters breaking' turned out to be nothing more than some rather severe urinary incontinence. To this day, I am still amused and quietly giggle at this scenario, even though I know I shouldn't, because I could very well make the same sort of mistake. I was getting an incredible amount of discharge during my pregnancy and genuinely felt like I wee'd my pants all day, every day.

'Sim, how do you know when your waters have broken, is it obvious?' This was going to be Simone's second baby.

'Believe me,' Simone said, 'you'll know when it happens. It's a huge rush of water that will go right through your pants like a busted water balloon, not just a little squirt. Put some old towels in your car for the journey to the hospital; you'll probably need them.'

BUMP BOX:

Heartburn and baby's hair: is there a link?

Well, I'd always thought this was nothing but an old wives' tale. But interestingly, in 2006, a study (Costigan 2006) was conducted that proved otherwise.

It looked at 64 pregnant women, who each ranked the severity of their degree of heartburn during pregnancy, and then independent people dubbed 'coders' rated the amount of newborn hair.

Seventy-eight per cent of women involved in the study reported some degree of heartburn — with 23 out of the 28 women who reported 'moderate or severe heartburn' giving birth to babies with average or above average amounts of hair.

Conversely, ten out of the 12 women who reported experiencing no heartburn had babies with less than average or no hair at all.

The conclusion surprised the authors of the study: 'Contrary to expectations, it appears that an association between heartburn severity during pregnancy and newborn hair does exist.'

There you have it; hair and heartburn appear to be related.

For the record, I had no heartburn whatsoever throughout my pregnancy — and my baby was born with almost no hair.

WEEK 33
How did I become so mean?!

If I'd ever been nasty before pregnancy, well ... being pregnant was the Golden Ticket to Bitch Land where irrationality reigned supreme.

Case Study: How pregnancy turned this lady mean.

Husband and I always got takeaway on a Friday evening. He preferred Indian and I preferred Thai, but we were pretty good at taking it in turn.

This particular evening, we decided on Indian. We knew from previous experience the local curry house wasn't an option because they didn't make palak paneer (spinach curry with cottage cheese), which was my favourite Indian dish. And if we were going to have Indian, I wanted palak paneer.

As we hadn't lived in Logan for long (halfway between Brisbane and the Gold Coast), we did a quick internet search that revealed the nearest Indian place was about 15 minutes drive away. However, when we arrived, it was just a small takeaway style kiosk with bain-maries ... and none of them contained palak paneer.

I wanted palak paneer.

I felt if I had to have Husband's choice of takeout, I at least wanted the dish I liked best. I was absolutely ravenous, and it was already 8pm, but we got back in the car and searched for the next nearest Indian restaurant.

Because the next closest restaurant was on the other side of the highway — about a ten-minute drive away — and I was so very, very hungry, I thought I'd be smart and call ahead with our order and double check palak paneer was on their menu.

'Hello?' an old man answered.

'Hi, is this the Indian restaurant please?'

'No, they must have had this number years ago. I'm always getting calls. Did you want their number?'

'Yes, that would be great, thanks. Babe, type this into your phone.'

Husband called the number the old man gave us, placed our order (palak paneer and chicken red curry), and we drove to the address listed on the website. But when we arrived, there was no Indian restaurant, just an empty shop that used to be a dry cleaner and a KFC.

Husband phoned back.

'We're right behind the KFC,' the young counter girl told him.

After driving around for another five minutes, we physically got out of the car to look. Husband then needed to 'break the seal', as he'd been at the pub all afternoon and there was nowhere to go, so I had to drive around for another five minutes to find some dark bushes. Then we kept searching. By now they would have cooked our meal, and it would be getting either cold, or dry, or both.

'Why can't we fiiind it?' I wailed. 'Did you really need to

use the bathroom then; couldn't you have waited? I'm sooo *hungry.*'

'Geez, calm down, babe.'

'It's okay for you to say! You're half-pissed and haven't been driving around for 45 minutes with a pair of legs sticking into your ribs. It's NOT EASY driving when you're eight months pregnant. I'm *soooo* hungry. I give up. I can't drive anymore! Give me the damn phone and I'll call myself. You're really fucking this up!' I began to howl. The crying was so violent, I physically couldn't dial the number with my shaking fingers. I couldn't even see my phone. To be hungry and pregnant and to know there was food out there somewhere ... it was torture.

'Babe, this isn't good for you, and it isn't good for the baby. I haven't done anything wrong and you're being a cow.'

'Don't call me a cow! I'm not fat, I'm just fucking pregnant! Let's just go home. I don't want fucking Indian anyway.'

'Look, do you want me to drive? I feel fine.'

'Of course you can't drive, you've been drinking! You could kill us all! I have to drive, don't I? For goodness sake, if I don't get some food soon, I think I might pass out ... give me your phone and have the number ready to dial on the screen. Hurry up.' *Deep breaths, Mandy, deep breaths.* 'Hi. We ordered some Indian from you about half an hour ago and we are literally standing outside the KFC and can't see your restaurant anywhere,' I stated.

'That's strange,' she replied. 'If you walk behind them, where you can see their drive-through ordering window, you can't miss us.'

But they weren't there.

'Right, can you just give me your exact street address, so I can type it into Google maps again?'

'Of course. It's 32 Corban Street, Daisy Hill.

'Daisy Hill! That can't be right! We're at the KFC in Woodridge. Your website specifically says Woodridge!'

'Um ... I'm sorry, but we are in Daisy Hill. I'm not sure why it would say that; we've never been located on that side of the M1.'

I hung up the phone. 'NOOOOOOoooooo!' I was bawling. 'It's back where we started, 15 minutes back the other way! This is soooo messed up. I can't go on like ... like ... like at all!'

'Wow!' said Husband. 'That's amazing! What are the chances of having KFCs both where we thought it was, and where it actually was?'

In hindsight, I concede that was a rather interesting coincidence, but at that moment I was not in the mood for sharing a point of view with him.

'Who cares?! That's not helping! I just need to go home! Now!'

'Babe, you're hungry. We'll get the food. Just stop crying. We'll pick up our dinner and go home and start the evening over again.'

'This had better be the best fucking Indian I've ever eaten in my life,' I cried. 'Now direct me, and I don't want any mistakes or wrong turns.'

When we arrived, the restaurant had a totally different name to the Indian restaurant website I had looked up and thought I had phoned. Meaning, the old man had given me the number of AN Indian restaurant, but it mustn't have been the one that corresponded with the name and address of the phone number I'd called him on. *No way!*

While I was working out exactly how the mix-up had

happened, Husband had gone inside to collect our order.

'I explained to them about their website, babe, don't worry, they're going to fix the address online so it doesn't happen again.'

'Oh … but it wasn't them … oh actually … that's good … thanks.' I couldn't be bothered trying to explain the error properly, I just didn't have the energy.

So nearly two hours after we left to grab some quick takeaway down the road … it turns out the Indian place we eventually got our dinner from was only 12 minutes from our home.

Thankfully the curry was delicious, and slowly the colour started coming back into my face — the enormous chasm in my guts was satisfied and my brain cells eventually defeated my cray-cray cells.

'I'm sorry for being so dramatic, hon. I was just so hungry, and buying Indian shouldn't have been so hard. I'm so hormonal today. I shouldn't have taken it out on you. Thank you for being patient with me.'

'That's okay. Luckily, we're only living in this area for six months. There will be heaps of good Indian places to eat at once we move back to the Gold Coast.'

BUMP BOX:

What you want to hear at 33-weeks pregnant.

If anyone is having difficulty dealing with your mood swings, please show them this list of things they should be saying to you, in order to cheer you up:

- 'Your glow is so amazing the entire world wants to rub their faces under your armpits and use your sweat as a youth serum.'
- 'You're so productive — is that bump secretly hiding a solar panel?'
- 'Of course I don't mind if we stop for the bathroom again; I love being late!'
- 'What excess fluid? I thought you'd just had filler in your ankles; they look amazing.'

Of course, feel free to come up with some of your own!

WEEK 34
Crossing Biffin's Bridge.

If a guy asks you whether he can cross Biffin's Bridge, he is not, I repeat not, asking for directions to the nearest river. Your perineum — also known as your Biffin Bridge — is the area between your va-jay-jay and your bottom hole.

My doctor recommended I massage my perineum from 34 weeks right up until the main event, to give it a bit of a stretch. She said this was because during childbirth, the perineum needed to stretch in order for the baby's head to fit through the vagina — and apparently massaging the perineum (i.e. giving it a stretch) can lessen the risk of tearing during childbirth.

As I began the massage, I immediately felt a burning sensation Down There, like rubbing Deep Heat into my gums. (Not that I've tried eating Deep Heat, but I'm pretty sure it would feel something like this did.) One of the main reasons my doctor recommended the massage was to give me a taste of the burning sensation before the birth; she said I'd feel the same sensation when my baby's head came through my vagina. (In retrospect, my doctor was right about this; I knew what to expect and it did make the pain more palatable for me.)

Massaging my Biffin Bridge felt very unnatural, sort of like petting a dead fish. It also made my fingers smell like dead fish.

Apparently, some women ask their partners to massage it for them; however, I was certain this was the only time my husband would explicitly say no to something fishing-related.

BUMP BOX:
Where is Biffin's Bridge?

Have you ever wondered why it's called a Biffin Bridge? The online community dictionary definition (Farlex 2021) describes it as 'The female perineum, that area of the anatomy between the vagina and the anus where the male testicles biff during copulation.'

People also refer to this skin as the 'taint', the 'gooch' or the 'grundle'. Who says you don't learn something new every day?

WEEK 35
Weeing my pants ... it happened!

I had just finished a long day at the office, mustered the energy to walk Captain around the block and came back inside to look at the clock. 7pm. It was getting late. Husband was out of town.

My stomach moaned, and I bent my stiff fingers, willing them to warm up enough to cook some comfort food. *What's for dinner?* I thought. *Something quick and easy. spaghetti bolognese. Better start chopping that onion. But I haven't been to the bathroom in almost two hours, and I really need to pee. I'll just get that onion browning. I'm so very hungry.*

Then ... *AHHHH-CHOO!* Wee slam-dunked into my undies. The urine did not pass Go; it did not collect $200. It happened without my permission, without any prior warning and shocked me to my ever-weakening core.

As the stream of urine started running down my leg, I reached down to my knees and frantically wiped in an upward motion, as if I could scoop the wee up and push it back through my pants into my urethra. Did this really just happen? I needed to pretend this wasn't happening. I was embarrassed enough when it happened alone in my own home just now; what if I sneezed at work or when I was out with friends?

From my fingers right down to my toes, I was covered in

urine. I wanted to laugh but I was so exhausted I could only cry. I was torn between cleaning myself or cleaning up the floor first; the former would mean I potentially dripped wee through the house, the latter meant I stayed covered in urine for another five minutes. Neither option was appealing.

This, I thought, *means I haven't been practising bracing my pelvic floor enough.* I saw my future flash inside my mind. *I'm a total failure to myself, so I'll probably fail as a mother. This means my child will end up on benefits and refuse to wear shoes. I'll spend my superannuation buying her a house to live in, and she'll set it on fire with a toaster. But I won't notice, since I'll be broke and living in the basement, while she throws scraps of food to me like a dog.*

I was wailing in disgust but unable to wipe away my tears of devastation, due to the whole urine-on-my-hands thing.

I decided a long, soothing shower would be best. Then I walked back to the kitchen, ignoring the drops of wee on the floor, and instead buttered some toast.

It tasted incredible.

Don't be upset if you can't cook the spaghetti; some days you're only meant to eat toast. Remember those words. I found them useful, not only throughout the rest of my pregnancy, but also the rest of my life.

BUMP BOX:
What's the definition?

'PEEZE: noun — a sneeze that results in peeing your pants.' (Urban Dictionary 2015)

WEEK 36
Is Baby Brain real?

Moving house while pregnant is not a good idea for many reasons. Oh — have I mentioned this before? I was delving back into the laborious, time-consuming, yet-oh-so-cleansing mission, all in the name of moving back to where I had always imagined myself bringing up babies: the beachside city of the Gold Coast.

After our last experience, the mere thought of moving house at 36 weeks pregnant was enough to put me into early labour.

To make matters worse, I'd been so busy winding up my job and doing a handover, it had taken me by complete surprise to find out our current lease was up in exactly eight days time. The entirety of which Husband was going to be working on the other side of the state. This meant I'd need a well-oiled plan, namely:

- three days to pack (not easy, given I had the mobility of a Telly Tubby)
- day four, for the movers to collect our things
- day five, for the bond cleaners to clean
- day six, to have the carpets cleaned and pest control done
- two spare days as a contingency.

Except … I had somehow forgotten to find us somewhere else to live. I'd been sure it was still at least another month away! This was 100 per cent uncharacteristically unorganised of me, which led me to the conclusion that Baby Brain was a real thing.

With my bowling ball strapped to my front, I spent the next few days driving the hour-and-a-half round trip to and from the Gold Coast, plus countless hours driving in between houses once I got there. The Gold Coast rental market was overpriced and fiercely competitive, with usually at least a dozen other potential tenants at the inspections. I traipsed through what felt like a trillion rentals, none of which were remotely suitable because they looked nothing like they did online.

Photos of the rooms had obviously been stretched to make shoeboxes appear like ballrooms, and I'm sure the paint job at one house was done several years before the photos were taken, because I didn't recall seeing 'Dave's not coming home today or eva' graffitied in the hallway in the advert. (Which I decided to give the house points for, since Dave didn't sound like someone I wanted to meet.)

During those viewings, I found one house that could have been classed as 'nice'. The others fell into the 'rotten', 'smelly' or 'Captain would have nowhere to go to the toilet' categories. (When did people stop having backyards in Australia?)

Of course, the 'nice' house inspection was packed full of ambitious soon-to-be-homeless people like me. One potential tenant followed the property manager around the house saying things such as, 'My husband just got a huge promotion' and 'My Salvia Phyllis Fancy plant would look absolutely fabulous in that corner' and 'What gorgeous shoes you're wearing, you have to tell me where you got them!' It dawned on me I needed to up my game if I was going to secure a house within my short timeframe.

Being visibly pregnant was somewhat helpful. It was sort of like holding a giant sign over my head saying 'Nope, no parties at my house for a while!' However, after finding out how competitive the rental market was, I felt like I needed something more ... something that would *really* seal the deal. But what? I racked my brain but no cigar. Little did I know fate would intervene ...

Following a disappointing day of house-hunting, I tried to clear my head by taking Captain for a walk. Mind you, he was a bouncing brute weighing 47 kilograms, and I was eight months pregnant with the muscle tone of a jellyfish, so you can imagine who really walked whom.

Anyway, I often took Captain to a clearing down the road that was large enough for me to let him off his lead and give him a good run around. There was a small hill at one end, and Captain often sat on top of the hill, smiling and inspecting his surroundings like he was King of All Hot Diggety Dawgs, as drool cascaded down from his jowls. *Let's give him a solid bit of exercise, I thought. It'd be great to have him run up and down the hill.*

I stood at the bottom of the hill. 'Captaaain! Come here, buddy! Come on!'

Husband had this game he played with Captain, whereby when our dog galloped towards him, Husband would jump in the air making an arch with his legs and allowed Captain to run through underneath it. This was IMPORTANT INFORMATION.

I should have remembered this IMPORTANT INFORMATION, but you know, Baby Brain. Captain bounded down the hill and came at me full pelt, grinning from ear to floppy ear.

I don't really recall what happened next — where he hit me, what was going through my mind, or exactly how I landed. But I do remember both of my legs disappeared for a moment, then I couldn't get up off the ground due to the lack of air in my lungs. I remember waiting for the searing pain in my back to go away, but it didn't. I lay on my back for at least 15 minutes, while a panting, contented Captain sunned himself beside me, oblivious to my pain and obviously quite pleased with how the 'game' had gone.

Once I ascertained which way was up, naturally my next thought was for the baby. *I'm not the first pregnant woman to be knocked over, and I certainly won't be the last,* I thought. *I landed on my back, not my stomach. Actually, that could probably still cause some real problems for our baby. OMG, this is it. Our baby is going to have curvature of the spine. Or brain damage. Did I knock the placenta loose? Is our baby still breathing? Why can't I feel the baby moving? Shit shit shit!!!*

I lay there in shock, crying. Eventually I realised cars driving past couldn't see me because of the hill, and I was going to have to either help myself up or lie there until I pooped my pants and there was a westerly breeze and the stench eventually gave my position away.

In excruciating pain, I managed to limp the 100-metre walk home, though it took about 20 minutes. During this time, Captain figured out I was genuinely very sore, and he walked slowly beside me, occasionally giving me a sympathetic look as if to say, 'Mum, I liked winning and all, but maybe next time I should just play with Dad, huh?'

I gingerly lay on the couch, my back still feeling tremendously painful, and called the hospital. The midwife I spoke to said if I wasn't cramping or bleeding and the baby was still moving, we were both most likely fine. After a few minutes, I felt a surge of relief as the familiar butterfly feeling twittered through my stomach. Husband was hundreds of kilometres away with work and I didn't want to worry him, so I ran myself a hot bath, then tried to sit down and relax, but alas, sitting on a hard surface was impossible due to the hot pain in my lower back. This was not good. I was going to need a crutch to get around.

Then I remembered tomorrow's Open Home.

Pregnant AND injured? That would have to pull at some agent's heart strings.

We got the house. And we paid someone else to do all the moving.

BUMP BOX:

Baby Brain uncovered.

In a nutshell, yes, Baby Brain exists. Research released by Deakin University (Davis, 2018) has proven it really does exist; however, the scientists say more studies are needed.

The researchers examined information from 20 studies, including 709 pregnant and 521 non-pregnant women, which revealed women do experience what's scientifically defined as 'cognitive changes' during pregnancy. Symptoms of the Baby Brain phenomenon are known to include poor concentration and absentmindedness.

The analysis revealed the general cognitive, memory, and executive functioning performance of pregnant women was significantly lower than in non-pregnant women, both overall and particularly during the third trimester of pregnancy.

Lead researcher Sasha Davies, a PhD candidate in the School of Psychology, said it was important to note there were limitations to the available data used in the study — for example, other factors that could impact a person's memory, such as having multiple children, weren't accounted for.

Deakin University is conducting subsequent research to shed more light on the topic.

WEEK 37
Getting to the bottom of the poop problem.

Pre-pregnancy, my mind's eye already knew exactly how my pregnancy would look. I would stand on a clifftop at sunset, the wind caressing my hair, and a billowy white dress would sail gracefully around my smooth, round belly. Relaxing music would play as a peaceful smile rested upon my face, then I'd sweetly look down at my bump and sparkle with joy. Of course, there would be a photographer present to catch these special moments.

Funnily enough, at no point did this image involve small amounts of green poop stuck to my undies (and obviously, these ghastly little lumps would have been visible in my near-sheer dress).

It was like the Soviet Union was using my anus as a testing ground for nuclear weapons. During the last few weeks of my pregnancy, my bottom BURNED for anywhere up to 30 minutes following a bowel movement. And these were not your bog-standard bogs. Sticky, green and smelly, plus difficult to push out, they tagged the sides of toilet bowls like inkblot pictures at the psychiatrist. The similar proportions of gentleness and elbow grease required before finishing the job couldn't guarantee I was totally clean, so I often had to bend over naked in front of the mirror. (By this stage my little leprechaun friend was missing a couple of fingers.)

One day, after a fourth-round battle with the toilet, I limped back to my desk like Blackbeard on his wooden leg and prayed that my ergonomically designed office chair would provide some relief. But alas, sitting down also meant less airflow for my heiney, so the longer I sat there, the hotter it burned.

I closed my eyes to stop the tears and grimaced while I waited for the pain to subside. For the first time in my life, I wished I owned a bidet. All I could do was breathe deeply and try to remain silent.

I was obviously a bit constipated, but I really didn't know what to do.

BUMP BOX:
Comprehending constipation.

Accredited Practicing Dietitian Tamara Parker said constipation could be an issue for some pregnant women.

'Changes to hormone levels (in particular progesterone) can lead to decreased movement through your digestive system,' she said.

'There is also a decrease in our water absorption, meaning stools can dry out and become harder to pass. Add to this the constipating effect from some vitamin supplements (iron and calcium, in particular) and decreased physical activity, it's no wonder over a third of women report constipation during their pregnancy. Constipation can increase nausea and result in

---

decreased intake of adequate nutrition, so it is important to make changes to support a healthy digestive system.'

Fortunately, a few simple dietary changes have the potential to help tremendously.

'My experience with pregnant women has shown that increasing dietary fibre through intake of fruits, vegetables, legumes, wholegrains and nuts and seeds can relieve their constipation,' Ms Parker said.

'Aim for two serves of fruit and five serves of vegetables each day, choose wholegrain breads, cereals and grains, and include legumes or nuts and seeds as an alternative to animal protein a couple times a week. Extra dietary fibre should be combined with extra fluids and daily movement. Aim for eight glasses of water and 30 minutes of low or moderate impact activity each day.'

Ms Parker said if constipation wasn't relieved by dietary or lifestyle changes, she'd recommend having a chat to your healthcare provider, who could suggest the most appropriate treatment.

WEEK 38
The signs of impending labour.

The Post-Pregnancy-Parts I'm looking forward to the most:
- Not farting in public.
- Not farting when I orgasm.
- Being able to pre-empt whether said fart will be loud or silent.
- Looking into my baby's eyes and hearing her gurgle.

The Post-Pregnancy-Parts I'm NOT looking forward to:
- People no longer offering to carry everything from a tic-tac to a table for me, because I shouldn't be doing that 'in my condition'.
- Getting even less than the pathetic six to seven hours of broken sleep I'm currently getting.

While I could hardly wait to go into labour, at the same time, I wanted to savour every last second of 'me time' before our baby arrived.

During week 38, my obstetrician did an internal examination to see where my cervix was at. The examination wasn't aimed at pinpointing an exact birth date, but more about giving Dr McDelivery, Husband and me an indication as to how 'ready' my body was for childbirth.

According to the exam, my cervix only had to dilate another ten per cent before I was baby-ready, but unfortunately, there was no way to pinpoint just how long that amount of dilation would take. I could be giving birth in three days or in two weeks, we just didn't know.

What I did know was I wanted at least another seven days of 'me time' before I went into labour. I wanted to stay in bed until noon. I wanted to eat ice-cream for breakfast. I wanted to go for long walks along the beach.

I'd never be able to have these days again, well, not for at least another 18 years.

Don't come yet, baby, I thought. *Words which, had they been spoken to my dear husband, could have avoided this whole thing entirely.*

I'd heard the word 'cervix' a million times by now. I'd seen one in a chart at the doctor. I'd even been the proud owner of a cervix for more than 30 years. But I still had to research information on the internet to understand exactly what one was. *Am I alone here?* (In case you are also wondering, the cervix looks a bit like a neck; it's the long, skinny passage that joins the uterus to the vagina.)

Recently, I'd started to feel something sharp poking me in the tummy; apparently these were 'twinges' in my cervix. I got them maybe two or three times a night once I'd settled onto the couch after a shower. Did these twinges mean my baby was coming soon?

I had no idea! Which lead me to wonder — and therefore search — what the heck ARE the signs of impending labour?

Three big signs of impending labour[1]:

Braxton Hicks contractions increasing in number: Braxton Hicks contractions are a tightening feeling some women get in their uterus during pregnancy. These 'contractions' happen sporadically, but if you notice them happening a lot more often, this could be a sign labour is a-comin'.

Your belly 'drops': Complete strangers would come up to me from around week 30 and say 'Oooh, look at you! Your belly is sitting really low; the little one must be almost ready to come out now!' and I would subsequently freak out. Then about two hours later someone else would come up to me and say, 'Oh, you're carrying so high! It must be a boy!' The takeaway from this is: Not even your obstetrician can tell you exactly when your baby is coming or the size it will be, so don't listen to random strangers.

But in a more literal sense, 'dropping' refers to when your baby's head literally 'drops' into your pelvis. This can potentially happen weeks — or just hours — before labour starts.

You 'unplugged': Unfortunately, this has nothing to do with the acoustic version of your favourite karaoke song. There's an enormous amount of mucus that seals your cervix closed while you're pregnant, which is called a 'plug'. This mucus must come out of your vagina before the baby does.

---

[1] I researched this extensively, both medical websites and general chat rooms, and the list was seemingly endless, so I have elaborated on the three signs that appeared most often in my searches

You might lose the plug in bits and pieces, or you might lose it all at once. Losing the 'plug' is sometimes called a Bloody Show, since blood is usually visible in the mucus. Once you lose your plug, you might well be about to go into labour. (Though not necessarily; sometimes women lose their plug days or even weeks before labour begins.)

In addition to the above signs, friends of mine have also reported a loss of appetite, diarrhoea, and bursts of energy right before they went into labour.

As yet, I'd had no signs I was aware of. I'd wake up every morning and literally the first thought I'd have would be, *I didn't have a baby last night. Phew. Time to chill today.* The next thought was usually, *Is it too early for ice-cream?* Followed by, *There's some beside my bed from last night; I could just drink it like a milkshake.* Concluding with, *I probably shouldn't do that given I'm pregnant. It'll taste sour. Where is Husband and can he take this bowl out of my sight before I do something Future Mandy regrets?*

This gave me another item to add to my 'Things I'm Not Looking Forward to Post-Pregnancy' list — Husband no longer waiting on me hand-and-foot.

BUMP BOX:

Is it a real contraction or Braxton Hicks?

The RANZCOG website (RANZCOG 2016) says Braxton Hicks are contractions which tone the uterus, but don't dilate (open) the cervix.

They occur throughout your pregnancy, but you may not feel them until the second trimester. Braxton Hicks may be quite strong and uncomfortable and are often called 'false labour'.

These contractions can be distinguished from 'real labour' because they disappear with a change of position or activity such as a warm bath or shower.

WEEK 39
Can acupuncture help baby be punctual?

Because I was 39 weeks and there were still no signs of a baby a-comin', I had to make a booking to be induced, just in case it came to that. (Note that 39 weeks isn't 'standard'; the timing will vary depending on where you choose to have your baby and whether your care provider deems induction appropriate.) Unfortunately, the only date left available in my obstetrician's diary sounded as appealing as giving birth in a pit full of snakes.

That date was ... *insert haunting music* ... Friday the 13th.

In my mind, having a baby naturally on the unluckiest day of the year was one thing, but *forcing* it to arrive that day was somehow much worse. I'm a little superstitious, and I absolutely resented the fact my baby could be born on one of the two days of the year nobody wanted to give birth — the other being Christmas Day. There were 365 days in a year, and I'd have been happy to give birth on 363 of them; was that too much to ask?

I started to look for the positives. I should be happy I can give birth in the first place. Mary-Kate and Ashley Olsen were born on Friday the 13th too, and they did okay for themselves. *Friday the 13th* was a very successful movie franchise, albeit very, very scary. (OMG, I did *not* want to be induced under any circumstances. Have you seen that movie?!)

Friday the 13th was regretfully pencilled into my diary, but I was determined to do everything in my power to convince my baby to arrive before then.

I'd heard of an old-fashioned induction method whereby one drank castor oil, but what exactly was castor oil anyway? Was it even safe? I didn't know whether to buy it from the supermarket (do you cook with it?), the pharmacy (or do you moisturise with it?) or Supercheap Auto (or is it the stuff you put in your car engine?), so I didn't entertain it and decided to give acupuncture a go instead.

I arrived at the clinic early one morning, half-expecting a woman wearing robes with no shoes to turn me away for having a nasty aura. Surely, it took a special kind of person to stick needles into another person for a living? But to my surprise, the room looked just like any other waiting room. The acupuncturist looked perfectly normal and more relaxed than a pair of yoga pants on Valium.

Her name was Gillian, and she was dressed in a floaty floral jacket and jeans, with tight curly hair to her shoulders. Her chill level was so off the charts, just hearing her say my name made me fall half to sleep.

'Maaaandy. So niiice to meet you. Come this way.'

I took off my jeans and hopped up onto the table in my t-shirt and undies. 'Is this going to be painful?'

'Not at all. Just a little sensation you may find uncomfortable for a very brief moment, but some people don't feel anything at all.'

'How does this work, exactly?' I asked.

'Your energy flows along your body in "energy lines" or "meridians", and we insert needles along specific points in these pathways, to stimulate certain parts of the body,' Gillian replied.

I barely felt a thing as the needles went in, and I was so relaxed I didn't even notice her leaving the room. I completely zoned out and fell asleep. Before I knew it, my half-hour was up, and after being un-needled, I somehow felt lighter both physically and mentally, so I figured the acupuncture had done *something*, though whether it would bring on labour was yet to be seen. My hospital induction was still nearly a week away, and I was told to make another acupuncture appointment for a few days time.

BUMP BOX:

Did my acupuncture result in labour?

I would say the results are inconclusive. Three days after the acupuncture, I went into labour. It was the 11th of June — my due date. Was this a coincidence? I really couldn't say for sure.

Perhaps my daughter, like me, was simply a stickler for being on time.

WEEK 40
What's in a star sign?

An article written by award-winning journalist David Marr and published in *The Sydney Morning Herald* (Marr 2009) described the results of a Nielson poll about Australians' beliefs. The poll found more than 40 per cent of us believed in astrology. And this statistic seemed even more significant when compared to the 34 per cent who believed in UFOs and the 22 per cent who believed in witches; clearly astrology is a 'thing'.

I'm certainly a believer in astrology. I don't live by my daily horoscope — I'm not quite that hardcore. But I can't recall ever meeting a person who didn't think their star sign's personality traits reflected their own personality to a certain degree. This was why I was concerned my daughter might not like me much.

Astrology tells me I'm a Taurus, which is represented by a bull. Taureans are meant to be down-to-earth, yet very stubborn. We traditionally also like expensive things and eat too much food. These traits all rang familiar to me.

My daughter would be born a Gemini, a sign representing 'the twins' or 'split personalities'.

Geminis were known to be incessantly curious, sparking the worry she'd have a million questions for me that I didn't have the answers to. Geminis are also quick-witted, so no doubt she'd be out-arguing me before she hit Prep.

To top it all off, my lovely daughter was being born during a Mercury retrograde, which meant she'd want to think and process information before she opened her mouth ... I can't even begin to relate to that. What if we had absolutely nothing in common?

Though in fairness to her, I say stuff like, 'it's not urgent-detergent', and my dance moves are literally a jazzed-up version of The Wiggles, so I should certainly hope she was going to be cooler than I was.

A Taurus mother and Gemini daughter were not listed as a good 'match' on any website I could find outlining the mother/child horoscope compatibility. Did we even have a hope of being friends?

BUMP BOX:

Do star signs impact your relationship with your child?

Penny Walters, Astrologer and birth chart expert, clarified this. She said star signs don't really impact the mother-child relationship, instead, they describe it. To better understand a mother-child relationship, we must look at both their birth charts.

'The birth chart is a map of the heavens at the moment of birth. It is this snapshot that describes the life ahead,' Ms Walters says. 'It also describes the mother-child relationship. The information you need to create the birth chart is the date of birth (including the year), place of birth (town or suburb) and time of birth (to the minute). When you get to know the different placements within each birth chart, you can better understand each person. [And] when you relate the birth charts, you can better understand the relationship and the impact each person has on each other.'

Ms Walters said I needn't worry so much about my star sign being 'incompatible' with my child, as there were many more opportunities to connect with her beyond our 'Sun signs'.

'I first need to explain that when we say our star sign is Taurus (or whatever it might be), we're actually saying the Sun was in Taurus at the moment of our birth. We also have a Moon sign, Venus sign, Mercury sign, Mars sign, plus several other signs! Each of these placements present an opportunity for connecting with your child and strengthening the relationship.

'It's actually very normal to see different connections between a parent and a child other than between Sun signs. For example, the Moon in the mother's birth chart may connect with the Sun in the child's chart. This connection could manifest as the child seeing the mother as a nurturing and supportive person in their life.

'Alternatively, Saturn in a parent's chart may connect with the child's Sun, and in this instance, the child would see the parent as someone who provides structure for them. It's a matter of relating the birth charts between the parent and child to find what astrological connections do exist (there will most likely be several!) and then working with these placements to encourage the best expression of these.'

Reading this made me more curious to meet my daughter and find out what sort of connections we'd create, and how they'd develop.

I didn't have to wait long.

WEEK 41
Popping my 'pregnancy virgin' cherry

11 June

7.30pm: I started having the occasional tight tummy cramp, like I used to the day before I got a period. Obviously, I wasn't about to be visiting Aunty Flo. Today was my due date. *Could this be it?*

8.30pm: *Argh! That cramp took my breath away. Maybe these were Braxton Hicks contractions?* I didn't want to make a fuss. Husband had had a massive day at work and was falling asleep on the couch, and even if this was the real deal, I thought he could probably get some sleep before I had to say anything. I'd heard labour could be more time consuming than building the Taj Mahal out of LEGO®, so I figured I'd wait and see how the next couple of hours played out.

8.50pm: *Faaaaark!* The next pain lasted for about 45 seconds. When I went to the bathroom, I noticed I'd lost more of my mucus plug, which had been progressively coming out throughout the day. *Side note: I was asked by a fellow pregnant friend how I knew it was my 'plug' as opposed to regular discharge mucus. Well, I knew it was my plug because there was enough mucus in my undies to grout my entire shower every time I went to pee.*

9.00pm: I stayed in the bathroom and called the hospital to ask one of the midwives whether she thought I was really in labour, since I honestly still thought these 'contractions' might just be fakies. Given I'd never been in labour before, how would I know?

'If the contractions are coming on regularly and getting closer in duration, you'll know you're in labour,' said the nurse. 'Once they start coming on five minutes apart, call us back and come on in.'

'We've just moved house, so we're living over an hour away on the Gold Coast — would that still give me plenty of time to get to Brisbane?' I asked.

'Sure, just give us a call before you come in.'

9.05pm: 'Who were you just speaking to?' asked Husband — I hadn't intended for him to hear me, but I guess it was unusual for me to be chatting to a friend in the bathroom at that time of night.

'Well, I've sort of been having these contractions — but they might not be real contractions or anything at all — so I just called the hospital to see what they thought.'

'And ... ?'

'Well, they said the contractions needed to be coming on regularly and five minutes apart before we can go in. At the moment, I've only had two and they were 20 minutes apart, so it might not be anything. They could be Braxton Hicks contractions.'

'Do they know we live more than an hour away?

'I told them. Anyway, we're both tired, let's go to bed.'

9.20pm: Another contraction. Followed by another, 15 minutes later. Then I had another one ten minutes after that, plus another one 15 minutes after that. In between the stronger contractions there were some weaker pains, but the midwife at the hospital had said to ignore those when I was timing myself. All my squirms and grunts were clearly keeping Husband awake, so I grabbed a spare blanket and slunk into the loungeroom.

10.03pm: *Hang on. Wasn't my last contraction only three minutes ago?*

10.05pm: *Another one two minutes later?!*

10.08pm: *Okay, I'm definitely not imagining this, my contractions are suddenly really close together now.*

10.10pm: *Eeek! What happened to five minutes apart?!!!*

I called the hospital again.

'Yes, you can come in now. We'll be expecting you.'

10.15pm: Husband walked groggily into the lounge room. 'I heard. Hospital?'

'Uh-huh. It's show time, baby.'

'Okay, then.' He dragged his feet back towards our bedroom, casually mumbled over his shoulder, 'I'm just going to grab a shower first. I need to wake up a bit.'

NOW? 'Oh. Okay. You know my contractions are only two minutes apart, right?' He either didn't hear or didn't understand the significance. *I guess I'd better eat a bowl of cereal or something. I could be in labour for days, and I hate being hungry.*

10.20pm: I sat down to my last supper as a childless woman: a bowl of Weet-Bix.

10.40.01pm: Husband emerged from the shower. 'I'd best go pack the car then?' he queried.

10.40.02pm: My waters burst all over the floor. 'Better grab a towel!' I exclaimed, as he simultaneously answered his own question. 'Yep!'

11pm: The car was packed, and we were on the road.

Thankfully, Husband had remembered to keep the petrol tank full. My contractions were still two minutes apart, but they were increasing in intensity. Every single squeeze to my uterus made it feel like an orange in a juicer, and with every agonising crush, another rush of water leaked through my tracksuit pants. Husband was driving 130km/hr down the motorway, while I stared at the ceiling and breathed deeply to stop myself from screaming.

11.50pm: Thanks to Husband's determination not to deliver the baby himself, the one hour 20-minute drive had only taken us 50 minutes.

'Why are babies always born in the early hours of the morning?' Husband lamented. 'Can't they come mid-afternoon? It's more civilised, then I can enjoy a beer after it.'

My brain pondered several warranted responses to this question — such as, *Shut the fuck up because if anyone will need a drink after this it's me* — but then another contraction hit, and I was unable to do anything but squeal.

12 June

12.00am: We were whisked away to the 'assessment suite', where a midwife ascertained I really was about to have a baby, then moved me to a birthing suite.

What was the point of that? I thought, looking down at my huge tummy and my sodden trackie dacks. *Were they going to send me to the broken arm department?*

The nurse told me I was five centimetres dilated, (which I supposed was the point of that), although I wondered where they sent women who were in labour and not as far dilated.

Then I stopped wondering anything at all that didn't involve DRUGS and WHERE DID THEY STASH THEM?

12.45am: A different midwife, a lovely lady around 50 years old with short grey hair cut very fashionably, said she'd be looking after me. She was called Elizabeth.

'What do you want for pain relief, dear?' she asked.

Great, I'd expected them to try and turn me off having drugs. 'I don't know that I want anything, I was just planning on seeing how I go,' I said. 'But seriously, does it get any more painful than this? Because if it does, I'm definitely going to need drugs. Like, I'm five centimetres dilated now, and I need to reach ten centimetres, so does that mean things are going to get twice as painful?'

'Everybody is different, and everybody's pain threshold is different. Why don't you give the gas a try, dear?'

'Because everyone says the gas is useless and doesn't do anything.'

'It might just take the edge off; it could be worth a try.'

Why not? I thought.

Elizabeth ran a warm double shower for me, so with my swimmers on, one showerhead on my back and the other on my belly, I kneeled and leant forward on a chair. Each time a contraction came on, I heaved heavily on the gas. *Wow. The gas felt gooooood. I was hiiiiiigh.* 'Baaaabe, this is soooo awesooooomee. You should tryyyy it,' I slurred.

In fact, I was so delirious, Husband asked the nurse, 'Should we turn the gas down a few notches?'

To which she whispered back, 'Don't tell your wife, but it's on the lowest setting.'

It didn't take *all* the pain away, and I can see why some people would rather an epidural, but for me it numbed the contractions enough to make them bearable, and it made my brain pleasantly mushy. Gripping the hose and breathing deeply also gave me something else to focus on when the pains were at their peak, and I felt kind of spacey and drunk in the meantime. *Oh, how good is this!* (Minus the sporadic cycles of agony.)

Around 1.45am: Before I knew it, it was time to hop onto the bed.

'Can I take the gas with me?' *Thank you, thank you.*

Swimmers off, hospital gown on. Game on.

Around 2.00am: I was on the bed. I was holding both thighs up to my shoulders as though modesty hadn't yet been invented. Between Elizabeth and Husband, I had a great cheer squad, coaxing me through every bit of pain. They kept telling me what great progress I was making, and I was 'almost there', but all I could think was *where's this freaking doctor then? I didn't pay to go private for her not to show up until the hard work is done!*

Obstetricians are wonderful people; I would even describe them as miracle workers, and I know they work ridiculous hours. But what if something went wrong? Why the heck wasn't there a doctor in my room? I guessed it may have been because my chosen obstetrician was on an RDO, so this poor other doctor had likely not scheduled me in.

Making me even more worried was the fact I had no idea which doctor I was getting, and I sincerely hoped it wasn't the one I'd read all the nasty internet reviews about.

'Where's the freaking doctor?' I kept yelling over and over, no doubt offending the midwife, and also giving Husband a sneak-peak of my 'Mum Voice'.

Around 2.30am: When the obstetrician finally did show up (thankfully it was an obstetrician I'd heard of before and had read great things about), I desperately wanted to grab her hand and stick it up my vagina and beg her to pull the baby out. I knew this wasn't exactly how they'd described the process in our antenatal class, but by this stage I was willing to try anything to hurry it along.

During each contraction, the doctor told me to push, then push again. And to keep pushing. Then, just when I'd run out of breath and my face was blue from the strain, she told me I had to push again 'and make this one count!' as if the other pushing had just been a dress rehearsal.

Around 2.35am: 'Oh no, I can't! I can't! No! No!'

The obstetrician grabbed my hand and forced it in between my legs, then made me tap on the crown of my baby's head. I was tapping on a blood-covered circle about seven centimetres in diameter as it protruded from my vagina. If that wasn't weird enough, the act was being reflected in a mirror being held by the midwife, so I could get a good view of it all. The baby's head was poking out of my lady hole like some kind of foreign object; it didn't seem to belong there. The last thing I wanted to do was touch it. But when you're in agony, high on gas, and your legs are propped up in the air, you have to take it as it comes.

'This will help, trust me,' the doctor said.

This wasn't the obstetrician's first delivery (thank goodness), and she was right about the mirror. Watching my reflection and touching the baby's head helped me give birth. I wanted to push as hard as I could. I wanted to get this baby out as quickly as possible. But seeing the baby's head gave me direction on how much to push and when to push and motivated me to push again, even when I was beyond the point of exhaustion.

With that confronting mirror being held up by the midwife, I could see things unfolding in all their glory. The pain was well and truly tearing me apart, though obviously nowhere near as much as it would have been sans gas.

When I started to lose patience with the pushing process, I thought about how lucky I was to even be able to give birth — there were so many women out there who couldn't conceive or carry their own child who'd give their right arm to feel the pain I was feeling at that moment.

The obstetrician told me once I started to feel the burning pain (that same pain I'd felt when I did the perineal massage), it meant I only had a few more pushes to go before the head would be through. And once the head was through, the body would follow naturally.

2.45am: It was overwhelming. It was wonderous. It was beautiful. Yes, it grazed my right labia and my haemorrhoids multiplied like Viagra-laden rabbits, but the people ain't lying when they say childbirth is all worth it. My vagina opened like an envelope at the Logies — with a huge amount of anticipation quickly followed by celebration — and I felt the pressure as my baby's head pushed through, then the rest of her body quickly followed. The head was the real stickler — to be honest, the rest just felt like a soft poop!

The look of wonder and joy on my husband's face alone was enough to melt me, but then I held my baby in my arms. My body was convulsing with the trauma of giving birth, so after being briefly enamoured, I handed her over to Husband, who cried and marvelled over who would undoubtedly become Daddy's Little Girl.

I thought it was all over, but then the doctor reminded me I still had to deliver the placenta, which was the icing on the exhaustion cake, but mercifully nowhere near as taxing as the birth itself.

Afterwards, Elizabeth stuck an anti-inflammatory up my

bottom to relieve the pain Down There, then I kept crying and shaking and staring at my husband and our daughter. It took 45 minutes for me to stop trembling from shock, then I could finally take our little girl back again and get a good look.

We'd decided to name her Indigo, because after nine months of arguing, it was literally the only name we both agreed on. She had wisps of dark hair (that would later turn white blonde), beautiful big blue eyes (that never changed), and a face reminiscent of her father's (that for the first few years constantly changed like a chameleon between her father's face, her grandmother's face and my face). Her lovely little nose was more squished up than I'd expected; no one had told me that about newborns! (Then I supposed if my face had been pressed up against someone's stomach for nine months, I wouldn't have a button nose either.) She was on the smaller side at six pounds 13 ounces, or 2.78 kilograms ('hardly worth having', as one of Mum's friends said). She was so fragile, I felt like if we held her the wrong way or too tightly, she might get squashed.

Husband and I were smitten. Regardless of anything else that had happened in the lead up to this moment — the arguments; the injuries; the sleepless nights; the embarrassing moments; the nauseating changes to my body; the pushing during labour causing every single capillary in my face to break, making me look like a traffic light — Husband and I looked at each other and knew it was all irrelevant.

Because we had done it. She had arrived. This amazing child was ours.

And we had absolutely no idea what to do with her.

We'd collectively held about three babies in our entire lives. I knew at that moment, no matter what pregnancy had thrown at me, it was going to be nothing compared to the challenge of raising this child.

Maybe that's why pregnancy goes for nine months; to start building our fortitude. Or maybe it's just to remind us that worthwhile things take time.

No one could have told me beforehand exactly what it would be like. Nothing could have prepared me for the extreme ups and downs. I still don't know everything about pregnancy, but I do know one thing for sure — it happened NOTHING like the way I'd imagined it in my head.

AFTER THE BIRTH

WEEK 42
Take the help, *all* the help!

'I didn't throw up or poo myself in there, did I?'

The following pause was so pregnant, I wondered whether we'd have to head back to the hospital.

'...You didn't throw up.'

'Oh.'

'You don't remember?'

'I was pretty out of it. It was a hard one, wasn't it? Or ... was it runny?'

'Um, they were stools. Can we talk about something else? I don't need to be reliving this.'

'You mean you didn't post it on social media?'

'Very funny.'

Damn. I should have known the Weet-Bix were a bad idea.

The first six weeks of parenthood could be a whole other book. At the hospital, I bled so hard I had to double-pack maternity pads into my black granny undies, and I could hardly walk.

The lovely nurses changed Indigo's nappy for me the whole time, so I had to get a crash-course in nappy changing right before I left. It turned out I couldn't breastfeed ... I took two breastfeeding classes at the hospital and saw two different lactation consultants, but unfortunately the severity of my inverted nipples combined with a low supply meant my baby was never going to be satisfied with what little she could get from me. I argued to keep trying, until one of the midwives finally said, 'Listen to your baby crying. It's starving. It won't stop crying if you don't give it some formula.' So, I pumped what little breast milk I was getting and topped her up with formula supplied by the hospital. I was disappointed, but not overly surprised.

We had visitors at the hospital, but I was so busy doing various classes and trying to feed my baby and attempting to get sleep, the visits were rather rushed (though appreciated). I met other mums who had cut the rush to the hospital finer than us; one mum went into labour at 4.30pm, arrived at the hospital at 5.30pm and had the baby at 5.35pm!

When we got home, I thought I'd not want any help. I wanted to prove I was the best mother and didn't need any help; boy was I wrong! TAKE THE HELP.

There were moments I couldn't get my baby to sleep; there were days I didn't have a chance to brush my teeth until 2pm; there were days I'd call my husband in tears and tell him I hated our child because she wouldn't stop crying and I didn't know why. There were times she pooped while I was changing her nappy and the ghastly, smelly brown poop spurted like volcano lava across the room, decorating the new nursery rug, feeding chair and wall like a Jackson Pollack painting. I collapsed with relief when my mother arrived to help during the second week.

Husband had gone away with work, and I was all on my own and not coping.

Seriously, a love child between MacGyver and a scout leader would struggle to prepare for this. I've never felt as clueless in my life as the first few weeks of joining the mamahood — even more clueless than I felt during my first pregnancy.

Here are just a few of the challenges provided by my new bundle of joy:

1. While I was pregnant, I used to whinge about only getting five hours of broken sleep; this I now considered a sleeping marathon.

2. Due to severe sleep deprivation, I couldn't remember simple things like whether I showered that morning or whether I'd last pumped my right or left breast.

3. My baby would be screaming for half an hour before I realised I hadn't checked the nappy. But then I only changed it five minutes ago, didn't I? I seriously couldn't remember.

4. When I went to change the nappy, I forgot to fold out the frilly bits around the legs, meaning the next poop went all through my baby's new white leggings, onto the muslin wrap and onto my jeans. Once I took the nappy off, Indigo would manage to stick her foot into the poop. While trying to clean her foot, I'd get poop on my finger. Then I'd touch the change table and the cot, turning the nursery into a Tiny Poop Town.

5. Stretching a little singlet hole over my baby's comparatively large head became a complex physics assignment.

6. My baby cried, I stuck the dummy in. The baby spat the

dummy out. I stuck the dummy in. The baby spat it out. This continued until I gave up and put the baby into bed with me, so she would be quiet. Indigo: 1. Me: 0.

7. I thought my baby was smiling because she was happy, thanks to my amazing parenting skills. Wiser friends informed me she was far too young to smile and that look on her face simply meant a fart/shart/burp/spew was imminent. They were right.

8. I used to have time to keep up with current affairs by reading the paper and watching the news. Now I wished someone would invent nappies with the front pages of the newspaper printed on them, because it's the only way I'd find out a miniature tornado ripped apart the house next door yesterday.

9. Indigo usually looked sweet and adorable, so I turned down offers to look after her. A few hours later, the screaming devil-child wouldn't shut up, and I wished I'd taken up the babysitting offer so I could go shopping/to the bar/to get a pedicure/visit the Bahamas for the next three months. TAKE THE HELP.

10. My baby woke every 40 minutes to two hours. So, after six weeks of being exhausted beyond belief, I called a Sleep Consultant who came to my home, showed me how to make my baby sleep and changed my life nearly as much as having the baby in the first place.

Though it wasn't all doom and despair — between the insanity and confusion and tiredness, there was love, laughter and hope. There were quiet moments at 2am when it was just her and me, smiling at each other. There was Daddy tickling her tummy. There were family photos and walks along the beach; Husband and I listening to her every sound and trying to memorise her every facial expression.

It took me nine months to work it out, but I realised I'd worried for nothing.

My pregnancy had been better than I could have ever expected. My pregnancy *was* the best. It was the best because it was mine. It belonged to me and produced a beautiful child, and whatever happened before this moment, it really didn't matter anymore.

ACKNOWLEDGEMENTS

For all the women who have struggled with fertility, I see you and I feel for you. While I can never understand your struggle, I hope your story has a happy ending.

For my parents, thank you for bringing me into this world and raising me to be an emotional human being, gifting me a love of reading, and beautifully preparing me to raise a family of my own.

For Husband, thank you for allowing me the time to write in peace, and of course, for getting me pregnant in the first place.

Family and friends who asked about this project of mine and continued to be supportive, your belief buoyed me in ways you'll never know.

Huge gratitude to all of my friends who agreed for their stories to be shared in this book — you know who you are.

Esther and John, I am so appreciative of the countless hours you spent babysitting while I tapped away at my computer (even though I know you loved doing it).

To Kit Carstairs, I may have written the book, but you made it sparkle! Thank you for understanding me and what I was trying to create.

Thank you to the following people/organisations: Katrina Dang, Shariqa Mestroni, Dr Alexandra George, Arts Law, Endometriosis Australia, Optometry Australia, the Australian Dental Association, the Royal Australian New Zealand College of Obstetrics and Gynaecology (RANZCOG), The National Health and Medical Research Council, Baby Center Australia,

Pregnancy, Birth and Baby, Parents.com, the Australian Breastfeeding Association, Dr Cathy Reid, Deakin University, The Women's Hospital, Samantha Costa, The Western Australian Department of Health, Fair Work Australia, Perinatal Anxiety and Depression Australia (PANDA), the Queensland Nurses and Midwives Union, Penny Walters, Tamara Parker, Dr Emma Black, Sandy Mocnike, and all of my beta readers — without your generosity, this book wouldn't be.

Finally, thank you to all the mums-to-be who read this book. Pregnancy is a crazy ride; I hope sharing in my experience has helped you in some small way.

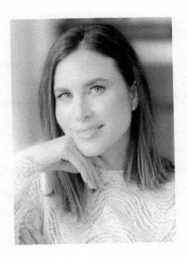

Mandy Mauloni is an author and freelance writer who lives on the Gold Coast, Australia.

She's previously worked in television journalism and production, as well as political public relations.

She enjoys spending time with her young family, eating Freddo Frogs, wearing toe socks, and marvelling at sunsets.

Find out more at www.mandymauloni.com

SOURCES

1. BabyCentre 1997–2021, *What cervical mucus looks like: photos*, BabyCentre, L.L.C, viewed 3 November 2020, <https://www.baby center.com.au/l1047500/what-cervical-mucus-looks-like-photos>

2. Costa S, 2019, Queensland Fertility Group, *Warning about the accuracy of fertility apps used by thousands of women to help in baby making*, QFG, viewed 5 May 2021, <https://www.qfg.com.au /about-us/media-releases/warning-about-the-accuracy-of-fertility-apps-used-by-thousands-of-women-to-help-in-baby-making>

3. Healthy WA 2021, *Morning sickness*, Department of Health, Government of Western Australia, viewed 10 March 2021, <https://healthywa.wa.gov.au/Articles/J_M/Morning-sickness>

4. The Royal Australian and New Zealand College of Obstetricians and Gynaecologists 2016, *Exercise During Pregnancy*, RANZCOG, viewed 3 March 2012, <https://ranzcog.edu.au/RANZCOG_SITE/ media/RANZCOG-MEDIA/Women%27s%20Health/Patient%20 information/Exercise-during-pregnancy-pamphlet.pdf?ext=.pdf>

5. Pregnancy Birth and Baby 2020, Vaginal discharge during pregnancy, Health Direct Australia, viewed 29 January 2021, <https://www.pregnancybirthbaby.org.au/vaginal-discharge-during-pregnancy>

6. Fair Work Ombudsman 2009, *Pregnant employee entitlements*, Australian Government, viewed 25 November 2020, <https://www.fairwork.gov.au/leave/maternity-and-parental-leave/pregnant-employee-entitlements>

7. The Royal Australian and New Zealand College of Obstetricians and Gynaecologists 2020, *Food to avoid*, RANZCOG, viewed 3 March

2021, <https://ranzcog.edu.au/RANZCOG_SITE/media/RANZCOG-MEDIA/Women%27s%20Health/Statement%20and%20guidelines/Clinical-Obstetrics/Common-Questions-in-Pregnancy-2020-V2_1.pdf?ext=.pdf>

8. *NIPT information.* Queensland Nurses and Midwives Union 2021, Quotations provided by email, received 10 August 2021.

9. *Dental health information.* Australian Dental Association 2021, Quotations provided by email, received 24 February 2021.

10. Parents.com 2015, *Is it normal to have weird dreams during pregnancy?* Meredith Corporation, viewed 1 December 2020, <https://www.parents.com/pregnancy/my-body/is-it-normal-to-have-weird-dreams-during-pregnancy>

11. Black E, 2020, Gender Disappointment in Pregnancy, Dr Emma Black, Clinical Psychologist, viewed 17 March 2021, <https://townsvillepsychologist.com.au/gender-disappointment>.

12. PANDA 2017, *Loss and grief during pregnancy*, Perinatal Anxiety and Depression Australia, viewed 24 March 2021, <https://www.panda.org.au/info-support/during-pregnancy/adjusting-to-change/loss-and-grief>

13. James J, 2020, Maternal caffeine consumption and pregnancy outcomes: a narrative review with implications for advice to mothers and mothers-to-be, PubMed.gov, viewed 29 May 2020, <https://pubmed.ncbi.nlm.nih.gov/32843532/>

14. National Health and Medical Research Council 2020, *Australian Guidelines to reduce risk from drinking alcohol*, Australian Government, viewed 11 May 2021, <https://www.nhmrc.gov.au/health-advice/alcohol>

15. The Royal Australian and New Zealand College of Obstetricians and Gynaecologists 2020, *Skin and Hair Care*, RANZCOG, viewed 5 March 2021, <https://ranzcog.edu.au/RANZCOG_SITE/media/

RANZCOG-MEDIA/Women%27s%20Health/Statement%20and
%20guidelines/Clinical-Obstetrics/Common-Questions-in-
Pregnancy-2020-V2_1.pdf?ext=.pdf>

16. *Milk ducts information.* The Australian Breastfeeding Association 2021. Research by Ramsay et al provided by email, received 7 September 2021.

17. The Women's n.d., *Premenstrual conditions*, The Royal Women's Hospital, Victoria, Australia, viewed 11 March 2021, <https://www. thewomens.org.au/health-information/periods/periods-overview/premenstrual-conditions>

18. Endometriosis Australia 2021, Various quotations from website provided by email, received 7 January 2021, <https://www.endo metriosisaustralia.org/>

19. The Royal Australian and New Zealand College of Obstetricians and Gynaecologists 2020, *Weight gain*, RANZCOG, viewed 3 March 2021, <https://ranzcog.edu.au/RANZCOG_SITE/media/RANZCOG-MEDIA/Women%27s%20Health/Statement%20and%20guidelines/Cli nical-Obstetrics/Common-Questions-in-Pregnancy-2020-V2_1.pdf?ext=.pdf>

20. Koh S, 2020, *Is your contraceptive pill causing dry eyes?* Optometry Australia, viewed 11 February 2021, <https://goodvision forlife.com.au/2020/11/18/is-your-contraceptive-pill-causing-dry-eyes>

21. The Royal Australian and New Zealand College of Obstetricians and Gynaecologists 2019, *Gestational diabetes*, RANZCOG, viewed 6 March 2021, <https://ranzcog.edu.au/RANZCOG_SITE/media/RANZ COG-MEDIA/Women%27s%20Health/Patient%20information/ Gestational-Diabetes.pdf?ext=.pdf>

22. *Stretch marks information.* Australasian College of Dermatologists 2021. Information provided by phone call and subsequent email approval on 14 April, 2021.

23. Costigan, Sipsma, DiPietro 2006, *Pregnancy folklore revisited: The case of heartburn and hair*, PubMed.gov, viewed 25 May 2020, <https://pubmed.ncbi.nlm.nih.gov/17150070>

24. Farlex, Inc. 2021, *Community dictionary; information submitted by the users and not checked for accuracy*, Farlex, Inc., viewed 13 January 2021, <https://www.definition-of.com/biffin+bridge>

25. Davis S, 2018, *'Baby brain' a scientific reality, but Deakin study seeks more data*, Deakin University, viewed 16 February 2021, <https://www.deakin.edu.au/about-deakin/news-and-media-releases/articles/baby-brain-a-scientific-reality,-but-deakin-study-seeks-more-data>

26. *Constipation in pregnancy information.* Accredited Practicing Dietician Tamara Parker. Information provided by email, received 18 April 2021.

27. The Royal Australian and New Zealand College of Obstetricians and Gynaecologists 2016, *Braxton Hicks*, RANZCOG, viewed 18 April 2021, <https://ranzcog.edu.au/RANZCOG_SITE/media/RANZCOG-MEDIA/Women%27s%20Health/Patient%20information/Labour-and-birth-pamphlet.pdf?ext=.pdf>

28. Marr D, 2009, *Faith: What Australians believe in*, The Sydney Morning Herald, viewed 3 December 2020, <https://www.smh.com.au/national/faith-what-australians-believe-in-20091218-l5qy.html>

29. *Star signs information.* Astrologer Penny Walters 2021. Information provided by email, 25 May 2021.

Printed in Australia
AUHW021227070322
360542AU00006B/12